The Female Mind:
A User's Guide

Edited by Kathryn M. Abel and
Rosalind Ramsay

RCPsych Publications

© The Royal College of Psychiatrists 2017

RCPsych Publications is an imprint of the Royal College of Psychiatrists,
21 Prescot Street, London E1 8BB
http://www.rcpsych.ac.uk

British Library Cataloguing-in-Publication Data.
A catalogue record for this book is available from the British Library.
ISBN 978-1-909726-80-2

Distributed in North America by Publishers Storage and Shipping Company.

The views presented in this book do not necessarily reflect those of the Royal College of Psychiatrists, and the publishers are not responsible for any error of omission or fact.

The Royal College of Psychiatrists is a charity registered in England and Wales (228636) and in Scotland (SC038369).

Printed by Bell & Bain Limited, Glasgow, UK

Acknowledgements

This book would not have happened without the commitment and vision of Deborah Hart, former Director of Communications and Policy at the Royal College of Psychiatrists, and Sally Dean, expert by experience. Deborah masterminded the book, the last of the trilogy of 'mind guides', in which mental health experts share their wisdom with a general readership.

Contents

Foreword

Until I reached my early 20s, I was happy to ignore the social realities of being a woman. As a child, I had an anxious temperament and I understood that a lot would be expected of me as an adult. It's no secret that the 21st-century woman is supposed to 'do it all'. On top of the career, relationships, babies and having the perfect body (cheers for that), women are also expected to be the caregivers, the domestic goddesses and the ones who remember everybody's birthdays. Never mind if you have the flu or your period is giving you grief, those plates mustn't stop spinning, and perish the thought that you drop one. I was intimidated, but thought that if other women could do it without complaint, then surely I could, too.

By the age of 24, that anxious 'temperament' of mine morphed into a full-blown anxiety disorder, eventually triggering a breakdown. I felt like a failure – everybody else seemed able to cope with life just fine, so what was wrong with me? I felt on edge constantly, tortured by panic attacks and bouts of insomnia. I was lost.

In my quest for knowledge about my condition, I devoured a great deal of reading material. Unfortunately, I only understood around 9% of what I read, and the dictionary became my best friend. The more I read, the more frustrated I became. It was all so complicated and scary. That's why I started my blog, *We're All Mad Here*, to write about mental health without the use of unexplained medical jargon.

In short, what I was looking for was this book.

I'll admit that when I was originally approached to write the foreword I rolled my eyes. 'Here we go again,' I thought, 'another stuffy academic textbook that only PhD students will understand'. However, within minutes of reading the first chapter I knew I was mistaken. *The Female Mind: A User's Guide* is a hugely important publication. It reads like a friendly guided tour of a woman's brain and covers a wide range of conditions. Basically, name it and it's there! There's even a fascinating chapter on the history of the female mind and gender inequalities. After reading Part 1, I felt revolutionised. Is it any wonder that women are more likely to develop some mental illnesses? We deal with a lot of rubbish!

Furthermore, this book is easy to understand. Hurrah! I can't believe there's finally a mental health book for the general reader – one that's interesting as well as informative.

Whether you're dealing with mental illness yourself, or caring for someone else, this book is for you. Packed full of information, case studies (called 'stories' here) and useful tips, it's a book you can dip in and out of, depending on your needs, or read in one go.

Hats off to the many authors; you're all fantastic and I wish *The Female Mind: A User's Guide* had been around 10 years ago.

Claire Eastham

Introduction: being female

What does it mean to be female? When we ask people this question, they all have an answer to it, in some form or another. And in some ways, we all know that the answer will depend on every individual's particular context or place in the world and, indeed, their age.

But never has there been a time when the question of sex or gender is more in play. Some people do not wish to describe their gender as female or male. We need to understand the meaning of new terms like 'gender fluidity' where a person likes to describe themselves as a mix of girl and boy, identifying differently depending on time and place.

By contrast perhaps, asexuality is used to describe a state in which sexual orientation is characterised by a persistent lack of sexual attraction towards any gender.

Given this change in the landscape from a simple binary idea of being female or being male, and of gender or sexual identity, you may well ask how we can poduce a book entitled *The Female Mind* with any degree of confidence.

We now know that being female is a very active process. In all mammals, the developing brain becomes actively masculinised so that the adult brain and adult reproductive behaviour are consistent with each other and with the sex cells (differentiated gonads) of the individual body. And although brain is thought of as being 'destined to be female' unless exposed to male hormones (testosterone) during pregnancy, we are now discovering that becoming female is not just a passive result of not having testes and not being exposed to testosterone. In fact, being female is a very active process indeed. To be female, the 'male genetic programme' has to be actively suppressed in females by a female-specific pattern of switching genes on and off by a process called methylation. Even more surprising perhaps, this brain feminisation is maintained by active suppression of masculinisation throughout life. More recent work suggests that this process can be influenced by a range of environmental effects (e.g. smoking/nutritional/ stress) to a greater or lesser extent.

What does it mean for mental health?

Being female is not just about brain. Sex differences in the perception of stress and the body's response to it have all been well documented and may in part explain some of the differences in rates of post-traumatic stress disorder (PTSD) and other anxiety-related difficulties. But, as we shall see in later chapters, being female (physically weaker and smaller) also means we have widely different experiences to men: greater poverty, less autonomy and power in the world, more suppression of desires, more sexual abuse and more inter-partner violence as a start. All these phenomena are likely to have an important influence on the female brain, as well as its behaviour, and to be responsible for some of the differences we see in rates of depression across women's lives. From a biological view, these negative life experiences act in much the same way as other environmental effects. And that's before we begin to consider the important socio-cultural, biological and psychological influences of periods, pregnancy or perimenopause.

We have invited a host of authors to cover all those topics, and more, in this book. We invite you to join us on this fascinating journey to discover – what is the female mind?

Kathryn M. Abel & Rosalind Ramsay

Part I.
Women in perspective

The history of the 'female mind'

Lisa Conlan

'The great question that has never been answered, and which I have not yet been able to answer, despite my thirty years of research into the feminine soul, is "What does a woman want?"' – Sigmund Freud (Jones, 1953)

Early mythology and theology

In classical Greek mythology, Pandora was the first woman. Zeus (king of the gods) created Pandora as a curse on man, a revenge on Prometheus for stealing fire from the Gods. Hesiod (750–650 BC), the Greek poet, gave us the earliest literary account: 'As fire's price I'll give an evil thing, which all shall cherish in their hearts, embracing their own scourge'. Pandora was given 'a dog-like, shameless mind and thieving ways' and, of course, her box, from which soon flowed all the evils of humanity.

In Christian theology, Eve was the first woman. Fashioned by God from Adam's rib, she was 'man's fatal partner' (Warner, 2001). All was happy in the garden of Eden until Eve enticed Adam into sin. After the 'fall' came exile, disease, mortality and hardship. From these beginnings emerge the founding myths of woman's place in Western history, told in a variety of forms: woman as original sin, created by and for man, and the weaker sex – morally, physically and psychically.

In the Middle Ages, the *Summa Theologica* by St Thomas Aquinas (1225–1274) was one of the most influential works of Christian philosophy. Woman were regarded as inferior to men, and the result of sin: 'as regards the individual nature, woman is defective and misbegotten' (Tasca *et al*, 2012). This text helped shape attitudes towards women and their capabilities for centuries, and its theological descriptions of woman's inferiority have been suggested as the start of a 'misogynistic crusade' in the late Middle Ages (Tasca *et al*, 2012).

Madness in the Middle Ages was either 'good' madness – exhibited by 'holy innocents, prophets, ascetics, and visionaries' (usually male) – or 'derangement' – seen as 'diabolic, schemed by Satan and spread by witches and heretics' (invariably female) (Porter, 2002). This attitude was exemplified by the witch hunts that spread through Europe, reaching their peak in the mid-17th century. They targeted women suspected of transgressing social, moral or behavioural norms, accusing them of sorcery and communing with the devil. Over 200 000 women were tortured and executed as a result (Porter, 2002). The enduring outcome was a culture that engaged in the widespread monitoring and vilification of 'abnormal' female behaviour.

> '...[Any] woman born with a great gift in the sixteenth century would certainly have gone crazed, shot herself, or ended her days in some lonely cottage outside the village, half witch, half wizard, feared and mocked at. For it needs little skill in psychology to be sure that a highly gifted girl who had tried to use her gift for poetry would have been so thwarted and hindered by other people, so tortured and pulled asunder by her own contrary instincts, that she must have lost her health and sanity to a certainty.'

So wrote Virginia Woolf (1929) in her seminal essay, *A Room of One's Own*. Writing from personal experience and in frustration, Woolf responded to what she saw as a patriarchal system designed to keep women subordinate and deprived of the rights and skills necessary to be free, creatively or otherwise.

It was a world where 'how to be a woman' was defined by men and what it was like to be a woman (i.e the female mind) was, frustratingly, the preserve of male 'expertise'. The history of the world has been told almost exclusively from the male point of view, serving the aims of men. Much the same problem exists in thinking about the 'female mind', perhaps better expressed as the condition of being a woman. This definition has been owned by men, from Genesis onwards. As Marina Warner (2001) notes, 'Adam is given the power to name Eve, make her his object and project meanings onto her'.

The 'female mind' was then understood as primitive, emotional and a biological fact (and failing) of being a woman. This distinction from the 'male mind' is seen in works such as Shakespeare's *Hamlet* (c. 1600), one of the most famous literary characterisations of madness. Hamlet, Prince of Denmark, exhibits melancholy resulting from intellect (or indeed may even, clever as he is, be playing at madness). Ophelia, on the other hand, descends into a chaotic, vulgar and emotional state of madness and is completely destroyed by it.

First approaches to mental health treatment

The Enlightenment (1650–1800) introduced the empirical, naturalistic paradigm of disease and the concept of man as a rational being. It was a time of great philosophical and scientific advances, bringing radical social reform and political change. 'Madness' was brought under the auspices of science, and taken out of the hands of the clergy and superstition.

The Victorian era saw a huge shift in attitudes toward the mentally ill and psychiatric treatment. Concerns about conditions for the mentally unwell, and poorly regulated madhouses across the country, meant that in 1808, England and Wales passed the County Asylums Act, mandating that every county must have an asylum in which the insane poor could receive treatment (Showalter, 1987). The asylums quickly filled up as demand outstripped supply. Shackles and brutal treatment were viewed as barbaric and the more humanistically oriented moral therapy was pioneered by the Quaker philanthropist William Tuke. At the same time, in Paris, Philippe Pinel (inventor of the bedside manner) was famously striking the chains from the mad of the Asylum de Bicêtre and La Salpêtrière hospital in an act of compassion, ringing in the new age (Appignanesi, 2009).

Despite these changes, the position of women remained much the same. They were viewed as inherently irrational and their 'natural' inferiority to men was later granted the status of scientific fact by Darwinism. In this model, women were confined to the roles of virtuous wife and mother. The excesses of the modern age, especially mental strain (i.e. education), were thought to cause particular physiological and moral imbalances in women and were strongly cautioned against by medical experts. Henry Maudsley, in his 1874 essay *Sex in Mind and Education*, regarded women as incapable of the intellectual work that came to men so naturally: 'when nature spends in one direction, she must economise in another direction'. This provoked a furious response from Elizabeth Garrett Anderson, the first female physician to qualify in Britain (in 1865). Such ideas were just as prevalent across the Atlantic, with Harvard's Edward Clarke writing that women risked physiological damage and infertility through proper education which would be 'neither fair to the girls nor to the race' (Clarke, 1884).

This situation did not, however, pass without criticism. Two of the most enduring literary works from that time, Henrik Ibsen's *A Doll's House* (1879) and Thomas Hardy's *Tess of the D'Urbervilles* (1891), were highly critical of the status quo and their heroines became emblematic of the hypocritical double-bind that Victorian society placed upon its women.

During the Victorian heyday of the asylums, there was a popular belief that female patients outnumbered male, but this was not the case (Appignanesi, 2009). However, there was substantial misuse of the idea of the 'madwoman', which was used to commit women who transgressed the social or sexual norms of the time, from illegitimate pregnancy to getting in the way of a second wife (Showalter, 1987; Appignanesi, 2009). This danger was very much alive in the imagination of Victorian England and was the subject of several notable literary works: *The Moonstone* by Wilkie Collins, *Cassandra* by Florence Nightingale and *Maria* by Mary Wollstonecraft. *Maria* was subtitled 'The wrongs of women' and described 'the misery and oppression, peculiar to women, that arise out of the partial laws and customs of society' (Showalter, 1987).

Michel Foucault challenged the idea that the Enlightenment had been a time of great improvement in the conditions of the mentally ill in his 1964 exposition *Madness and Civilization: A History of Insanity in the Age of Reason*. Instead, he dubbed this period the 'Great Confinement'. In his analysis, the Enlightenment had acted to silence and separate madness, stripping it of its previous spiritual worth and wisdom (as exemplified by characters like the Fool in *King Lear*). He proposed that the medical model created a false category, depriving madness of meaning and, as a consequence, dehumanising the mentally ill (Foucault, 1964). Foucault makes few references to women or gender, but his social constructionist critique of mental illness and his emphasis on the discourse of power have been influential in the feminist movement.

Jean-Martin Charcot (1825–1893), the famous neurologist of La Salpêtrière, is best remembered for his work on hysteria and hypnosis. La Salpêtrière was a huge institution housing almost 8000 women (1% of the total population of Paris) and was originally established to imprison prostitutes, debauched girls and female adulterers (Appignanesi & Forrester, 1992). Hysteria wasn't a new term (having been coined by Hippocrates to mean 'wandering womb'), but during this time it came to take on a very specific meaning and set of symptoms, rendering hysteria the 'female malady' *par excellence.*

Charcot believed that hysteria had a neurological basis and was due to a hereditary weakness, the key feature being extreme susceptibility to hypnosis. He studied and photographed his 'hysterics' with obsessive detail, and paraded them in front of huge public and medical audiences in what now seems like an exceptional piece of theatre. On stage, Charcot would use hypnosis to literally 'take control of the women's minds', and the women seemed compelled to do his bidding for the crowd, performing various degrading acts, such as stamping on imaginary snakes or kissing the hospital chaplain (Hustvedt, 2011). Although the witch hunts of the 17th century were no more in the 19th century, the misogyny behind them remained (Porter, 2002). The charge of witchcraft was replaced by that of hysteria.

A powerful symbolism emerges: man as puppet-master, creator of not just the acts, but the thoughts of women. Foucault was the inventor of the term 'medical gaze', which describes the power dynamic implicit in the doctor–patient relationship: a penetrating and objectifying gaze in which the doctor is party to a special and elite knowledge of the other, which he may or may not reveal (Foucault, 1973). The 'male gaze' was a term later coined by feminist film theorist Laura Mulvey to refer to the way cinema employs an almost unwavering central paradigm of the male subjective position, 'woman as image, man as bearer of the look' (Mulvey, 1975). Writer John Berger (1972) similarly identified this idea: *'men act* and *women appear.* Men look at women. Women watch themselves being looked at.' (p. 47)

Freud and women

Freud famously regarded women as a mystery, opening his lecture on the topic by saying, 'Throughout history people have knocked their head against the riddle of the nature of femininity. [...] Nor will *you* have escaped worrying over this problem – those of you who are men; to those of you are women this will not apply – you are yourselves the problem' (Freud, 1933).

As one of the most influential figures of the 20th century, Freud redefined the psyche and psychology and dramatically altered the landscape of our cultural lives. Alongside the concepts of the unconscious, mental conflict and repression, one of his central theories was the sexual drive theory of development. This was a phallocentric thesis in which women were re-cast as 'stunted men'. 'Women oppose change, receive passively, and add nothing of their own' (Freud, 1925). Almost 100 years later, this reads as little more than an extension of classical and religious conceptions of women, designed to maintain and legitimise the governing male status quo.

Freud's provocative theories of female sexuality and psyche have mostly been discarded, but a complex legacy remains. Feminist critiques of the 1960s were vicious, decrying his misogyny and patriarchal contempt of female sexuality, but modern readings are usually more generous, for there is a paradox at the heart of Freud's attitude towards women.

Freud was among the first to give voice to a previously unheard, oppressed group of women. He listened without judgement, faithfully recording the inner workings of women's minds in their own words. He recognised these 'hysterics' as intelligent and creative, and explicitly criticised the social and sexual restrictions of his time, blaming Victorian society for much of their unhappiness. In this way, Freud was radically progressive – even if he remained very much a Victorian man of his time. As psychoanalyst Hanna Segal (1991) said:

> 'I think Freud's theory that little girls think they have got the penis and then discover they don't is bunko. On the other hand, Freud was the first to treat women as human beings in the sense that he gave a proper place to female sexuality. He didn't consider them asexual beings. And even more important, I think, psychoanalysis is the first organized profession in which from the beginning women were treated exactly the same as men.'

It is worth remarking that it was a woman, Anna O, one of Freud's most famous patients (although he didn't actually analyse her on his own, but in collaboration with Josef Breuer), who was instrumental in originating his famous method of 'free association'. She suggested it as a technique that might help her to unlock the source of her misery (Breuer & Freud, 1895; Appignanesi & Forrester, 1992). Anna O, under her real name of Bertha Pappenheim, became an important social reformer and champion of women's rights. Appignanesi & Forrester (1992) point out that psychoanalysis came from women, and that without those that gave their time generously, there would have been no theory:

'from this vantage point, psychoanalysis, like feminism, emerges as a response to the "hysterical" women whose condition was emblematic of a collective malaise, and in turn a response to the untenable place of women in the late nineteenth century'.

Feminism

'Feminism has many mothers but only one father.' – John Stuart Mill (Reeves, 2007)

In 1869, against the background of a rising feminist movement, Mill published the essay *The Subjection of Women*, demanding an end to the oppression of women on moral and political grounds and passionately defending the right of women to vote (Mill, 1869).

Headed by Emmeline Pankhurst, the 'suffragettes' campaigned tirelessly to win the vote, along with simple social and property rights for women. After many failed bids to get even the most basic equality legislation through Parliament (the argument against was that women were too emotional and, as such, incapable of thinking as logically as men), the suffragettes turned to 'deeds, not words' (Purvis, 1995). They chained themselves to railings, set fire to postboxes, defaced Royal Mint coinage and even detonated bombs. A significant number were arrested and detained at HM Prison Holloway (Purvis, 1995). Refused their rightful recognition as political prisoners, many went on hunger strikes in protest and were subsequently force-fed. Women over 30 finally gained the right to vote in the UK in 1918, and this right was extended to women over 21 (the same age as for men) in 1928 (Crawford, 2001). In France, women won the right to vote in 1944. Astonishingly, Switzerland did not allow women to vote in national elections until as late as 1971.

Simone de Beauvoir published *The Second Sex* in 1949, ushering in second-wave feminism with her new and original distinction between sex and gender: 'one is not born, but rather becomes, a woman'. Quoting Kierkegaard, de Beauvoir begins, 'What a curse to be a woman!' It was unlike anything that had come before – the first historical and philosophical analysis of the radically asymmetrical relationship of women to men and their ordained inferiority. Anticipating the idea of the male gaze, she writes, 'she is the incidental, the inessential as opposed to the essential. He is the Subject, he is the Absolute – she is the Other' (de Beauvoir, 1949).

Literary critic Elaine Showalter (1987) examined the relationship between women, madness and psychiatry through the feminist lens in *The Female Malady*. Reviewing the previous 200 years, she saw the history of psychiatry as a power struggle between a patriarchal medical establishment and the women who were labelled 'mad' in a time when being female was increasingly pathologised. She describes a dual image of female insanity: 'madness as one of the wrongs of woman; madness as the essential feminine nature unveiling itself before scientific male rationality'.

Showalter also drew attention to the fact that, historically, more women than men received psychiatric diagnoses and institutional care. Andrew Scull, however, disputed this claim, suggesting that the difference amounted to no 'more than a few percent' and was more likely to be due to a greater reluctance to discharge women and their longer lifespan (Scull, 1989).

Women have also been disproportionately subjected to invasive treatments against their will, such as insulin coma, electroconvulsive therapy and frontal lobectomy. Showalter (1987) asked:

> 'But how should we interpret this fact? There have always been those who argued that women's high rate of mental disorder is a product of their social situation, both their confining roles as daughters, wives and mothers and their mistreatment by a male-dominated and possibly misogynistic profession [...] By far the most prevalent view, however, sees an equation between femininity and insanity that goes beyond statistical evidence or

the social condition of women [...] women, within our dualistic systems of language and representation, are typically situated on the side of irrationality, silence, nature and body, while men are situated on the side of reason, discourse, culture and mind.'

Here, the woman represents insanity. This is the archetypal image of the Victorian madwoman as exemplified by the operas, such as *Lucia di Lammermoor,* and the haunting, primal figure of Bertha Rochester trapped in the attic in Charlotte Bronte's *Jane Eyre* (Showalter, 1987).

The 1960s were a time of radical social change, with the rise of the civil rights movement, widespread feminism and antipsychiatry views. These movements challenged existing hierarchies and institutions, such as the idea of female biological inferiority and women's natural lower social status. Psychiatry's scientific status was also challenged, with prominent thinkers such as Thomas Szasz, David Cooper and R.D. Laing accusing psychiatry of misdescribing undesirable social behaviour as illness. Feminist writer Phyllis Chesler argued that, despite advances, little had changed in the relationship between women and psychiatry, with a dangerous conflation remaining between the two essential concepts of 'being a woman' and 'being mad'. In this way, female behaviours and attempts to transgress restrictive social norms were pathologised as 'penalties for being "female" as well as for desiring or daring not to be' (Chesler, 1972).

Conclusions

Today, there is no doubt that the situation for the Western woman has greatly improved. Increased equality and opportunity have made much possible that would have seemed inconceivable only 60 years ago. Women have increased social power and status to define and describe their own roles and experiences. However, there remains some way to go. Mental health, and its relationship with gender, is rarely out of the headlines.

Despite official figures from the World Health Organization (WHO) showing that rates of mental illness are identical for men and women, it remains true that women are twice as likely to develop depression or generalised anxiety disorder as men (Murray & Lopez, 1996). This difference, according to the WHO, is one of the most robust findings in psychiatric epidemiology (WHO, 2002). The archetypal gender disparity – neurosis and depression for women, substance misuse for men – is, unfortunately, borne out by epidemiological data (Freeman & Freeman, 2013).

What does it mean that rates of some psychological disorders are still strikingly higher in women than in men? The reasons for this are complex and under-researched, but the significantly higher social adversity faced by women compared with men remains a significant contributing factor (see Chapter 2).

Freeman & Freeman (2013) point to 'a toxic synergy between negative events, cultural values, and psychological and biological vulnerabilities'. Women's lives are harder. There remain inequality and gender asymmetry: compared with their male counterparts, modern women still experience increased social pressures, many more domestic responsibilities, more concerns with body image and reduced career opportunities, and, with these, increased levels of mental illness.

The history of the 'female mind' is the history of an idea as old as civilisation itself, created by and told for men: women as emotional, irrational and sinful. This idea has been culturally sanctioned, legislated and enforced by a patriarchal society. Those who dared transgress often paid a high price. Over the past 50 years, the emancipation of women and successive waves of feminist activism have significantly changed this narrative, but there remains a way to go.

References and further reading

Appignanesi L (2009) *Mad, Bad and Sad: A History of Women and the Mind Doctors*. W.W. Norton.

Appignanesi L, Forrester J (1992) *Freud's Women*. Weidenfeld & Nicholson.

Berger J (1972) *Ways of Seeing*. Penguin.

Breuer J, Freud S (1895) Studies on Hysteria. In *The Standard Edition of the Complete Psychological Works of Sigmund Freud* (ed J Strachey). Hogarth Press.

Chesler P (1972) *Women and Madness*. Palgrave MacMillan.

Clarke EH (1884) *Sex in Education*. James R. Osgood.

Crawford E (2001) *The Woman's Suffrage Movement: A Reference Guide, 1866–1928*. Routledge.

de Beauvoir S (1949) *The Second Sex*. Vintage.

Foucault M (1964) *Madness and Civilization: A History of Insanity in the Age of Reason*. Pantheon Books.

Foucault M (1973) *The Birth of the Clinic: An Archaeology of Medical Perception.* Routledge.

Freeman D, Freeman J (2013) *The Stressed Sex.* Oxford University Press.

Freud S (1925) Some psychical consequences of the anatomic distinction between the sexes. In *The Standard Edition of the Complete Psychological Works of Sigmund Freud* (ed J Strachey). Hogarth Press.

Freud S (1933) New introductory lectures in psychoanalysis. Lecture III: Femininity. In *The Standard Edition of the Complete Psychological Works of Sigmund Freud* (ed J Strachey). Hogarth Press.

Hustvedt A (2011) *Medical Muses: Hysteria in Nineteenth Century Paris.* W.W. Norton & Co.

Jones E (1953) *Sigmund Freud: Life and Work.* Anchor.

Maudsley H (1874) Sex in mind and education. *Fortnightly Review*, **15**, 582–594.

Mill JS (1869) *The Subjection of Women.* Longmans, Green, Reader & Dyer.

Mulvey L (1975) Visual pleasure and narrative cinema. *Screen*, **16**, 6–18.

Murray CJL, Lopez AD (eds) (1996) *The Global Burden of Disease: A Comprehensive Assessment of Mortality and Disability from Diseases, Injuries and Risk Factors in 1990 and Projected to 2020. Summary.* Harvard School of Public Health.

Porter R (2002) *Madness: A Brief History.* Oxford University Press.

Purvis J (1995) The prison experiences of the suffragettes in Edwardian Britain. *Women's History Review*, **4**, 103–133.

Reeves R (2007) *John Stuart Mill: Victorian Firebrand.* Atlantic.

Scull A (1989) *Social Order/Mental Disorder: Anglo-American Psychiatry in Historical Perspective.* Berkley.

Segal H (1991) *Women Analyze Women: in France, England and the United States* (eds EH Baruch, LJ Serrano). New York University Press.

Showalter E (1987) *The Female Malady: Women, Madness and English Culture, 1830–1980.* Virago.

Tasca C, Rapetti M, Carta MC, *et al* (2012) Women and hysteria in the history of mental health. *Clinical Practice and the Epidemiology of Mental Health*, **8**, 110–119.

Warner M (2001) *Monuments and Maidens: The Allegory of the Female Form.* University of California Press.

Woolf V (1929) *A Room of One's Own.* Penguin.

World Health Organization (2002) *Gender in Mental Health Research.* WHO.

CHAPTER 2

Gender-informed responses to women's distress

Jennie Williams and Gilli Watson

Karen's story

Karen is 27 years old and has been in close contact with mental health services since she was 13. She has been an in-patient for extended periods of time and has had four care coordinators in the past year. Karen was homeless prior to her last admission and will leave hospital when there is suitable accommodation for her.

Over the years, Karen has been variously diagnosed with borderline personality disorder, emotionally unstable personality disorder and psychosis. She has been treated with a range of medications, including antipsychotic medication. Staff call her 'attention seeking', as she often seeks support, though her named nurse describes her as 'muddled and confused'. Karen uses alcohol heavily and has been known to go missing from the ward, returning in a distressed state. Once, the clinical team was concerned that she might be pregnant. She self-harms frequently, often requiring treatment by accident and emergency (A&E) services; staff get frustrated and think this is a way of getting attention, describing her as 'manipulative'. Karen has difficulty sleeping and has confided in night staff that her voices tell her she is a bad person, a 'fat slag' who should harm herself and does not deserve to live. Karen says that she hates herself, feels she is being punished and that cutting herself gives some relief from the bad feelings and frightening voices.

Her physical health is poor; she eats badly and struggles to take care of herself. She has unstable diabetes, experiences frequent headaches and stomach pain, and asks staff repeatedly for medication.

Detailed information about Karen's earlier life is buried in her extensive records, and those staff who have gathered some of this knowledge are very uncertain about what to do to help; they don't give her opportunities to talk about difficult experiences she had, fearing this could add to her

14

distress. When Karen was a child, her stepfather sexually abused her over many years, which was known in her family; her attendance and attainment at school were poor; as a teenager she joined gangs where drinking and drug-taking were common. She became pregnant at 15 and her baby was given up for adoption – nothing is recorded about the baby's father and there is a possibility it was her stepfather's. The loss of her baby distresses her greatly; she only speaks about him after drinking heavily.

Most of Karen's male partners have been older men who have exploited her. It is likely she was raped recently when she stayed in a homeless shelter. Karen has never reported these abusive relationships to the police. She has no contact with her family. Friends she made while living in hostels also struggle with addictions and unstable, violent relationships. Karen wants to get well and then make contact with her son. She has never held paid employment, but has volunteered at an animal sanctuary and would like to work with animals.

Gender inequality, sexual abuse and women's mental health

Karen's story highlights the ways that women's efforts to survive lives that have been shaped by disadvantage and abuse can bring them into contact with mental health services. It also traces common ways that services fail to meet women's needs when this kind of information is unknown or not acted upon.

There is now a substantial body of research to support the conclusion that Karen's experiences are not exceptional. For example, there is convincing evidence that over half of all women using mental health services have experienced sexual abuse and violence, often severe and sustained. It is often also quite clear that those who have been impacted by these types of experiences are much more likely to be distressed and to receive a psychiatric diagnosis. People with histories of severe sexual abuse and violence are 15 times more likely to be diagnosed with 3 or more mental health disorders, to have attempted suicide, and are 12 times more likely to be admitted to a mental health in-patient unit.

Histories of abuse and violence predict disgnosis of depression, self-harm and diagnosis of borderline/emotionally unstable personality disorder, with early and severe abuse predicting the most severe difficulties. Childhood sexual abuse increases a woman's chances of experiencing auditory and visual hallucinations and of being diagnosed with a psychotic disorder. She is also at increased risk of other psychological and physical heath difficulties, including chronic pain, fibromyalgia, gynaecological and bladder problems, autoimmune difficulties and non-epileptic seizures. It is, therefore, concerning to know that the lives of young women appear to be becoming more difficult: a recent UK government survey finds that common psychological symptoms of distress and self-harming in young women aged 16–25 are significantly increasing.

Karen's efforts to survive the sustained, intentional abuse she suffered took place in a deeply gendered world, where women's and men's lives and experiences are still sharply differentiated. Gendered expectations mean that many women, like Karen, internalise the distress, shame and anger caused by multiple power abuses in ways that are gender congruent – hidden, often embodied, and typically harmful to themselves, not others. Using these strategies places women at high risk of contact with mental health services, Social Services and the criminal justice system.

In spite of convincing evidence that women's lives are disproportionately affected by abuse, trauma and adversity, mental health service responses remain medicalised and are slow to focus attention on the sources of women's distress. In many services the assumption that distressing feelings and harmful and difficult behaviours are symptoms of biological illness is still dominant. When this occurs, women experiencing serious psychological difficulties continue to be offered help which fails to meet their needs and can instead compound their difficulties. We suggest that it is essential to start with an accurate description of 'what has happened to her' and the origins of the difficulties she has experienced in gender and other social inequalities. The importance of this approach is that it rightfully identifies the reasons for her mental health difficulties in the adversity, abuse and trauma she has experienced and focuses attention on interventions that will address 'what has happened to her'. These interventions will not only empower her in her recovery and healing but also draw attention to what needs to change in women's lives and society in order to reduce women's mental health distress.

The importance of gender and trauma training for mental healthcare staff

When mental healthcare staff are not trained in trauma and gender inequalities, it is easy for them to assume that the strategies women develop to survive profoundly dangerous experiences are symptoms of disordered personalities, and to misdiagnose flashbacks and reliving of abuse as psychosis. Women also risk being judged and blamed for their difficulties. It is commonplace to hear staff describing women like Karen as 'attention-seeking' and 'manipulative'.

Health and social care staff need training to understand the broad effects of social inequalities on women's mental health, and the ways in which women's mental health difficulties are directly linked to strategies to survive abuse, multiple traumas, loss and deprivation. Staff need to feel confident that they can work safely and collaboratively with women to identify trauma and abuse. Women need access to trauma therapy services that can enable them to recover and establish safer futures. Fortunately, as we have noted, there is now a well-established body of theory, research and practice that can inform staff training, service development, and trauma therapy and recovery. Indeed, it is encouraging that a programme of 'trauma informed practice' training is currently being rolled out to staff working with women in prisons. This kind of training should be made available to all staff who have contact with vulnerable and disadvantaged girls and women.

We can rewrite Karen's story. For example, routine enquiries about abuse and violence in in-patient psychiatric services would identify her experience of sustained abuse and begin a trauma-informed understanding of her mental health difficulties. Her admission to psychiatric hospital and experience of homelessness could be averted through the provision of safe housing and support. This would also reduce the risk of further victimisation. Referral to community-based specialist psychological trauma therapies could begin her journey of healing and recovery; opportunities to network with other women survivors would help Karen establish safe interpersonal relationships and lessen her isolation, self-blame and shame. Finally, having a consistent care coordinator would provide stability and continuity and could enable Karen's referral to other health services, including diabetes, self-care and pain management to enable physical and mental health recovery.

References and further reading

Agenda: Alliance for Women and Girls at Risk (http://weareagenda.org/).

Cashmore J, Shackel R (2013) *The Long-Term Effects of Child Sexual Abuse* (Child Family Community Australia Paper No 11). Australian Institute of Family Studies.

National Institute for Health and Care Excellence (2014) *Domestic Violence and Abuse: Multi-Agency Working* (PH50). NICE.

NES (2017) *Transforming Psychological Trauma: A Knowledge and Skills Framework for the Scottish Workforce*. NHS Education for Scotland, Scottish Government.

Van der Kolk BA (2014) *The Body Keeps the Score: Mind, Brain and Body in the Transformation of Trauma*. Viking Press.

Female sexuality

David T. Evans

Evelyn's story

Evelyn was 80 years old. Her childhood sweetheart, life-long partner and soul mate – her husband – had recently died. I went to see her on a bereavement visit soon after the funeral. Evelyn invited me in and said there was something 'embarrassing' she needed to share with me, even more embarrassing given her generation and gender, and considering I was 30 and male. She tugged the leg of her trousers and said, 'I started wearing these before women generally wore trousers, before the Second World War. My parents beat me badly as a child; my legs are scarred so I don't like people seeing them'. Then she nudged me, smiled and winked and said 'My husband was always good to me – in the "bedroom department"'. But Evelyn's womb had dropped (her words), a uterine procidentia or prolapse, after her only child was born, and she had never told anyone in the 50 years since. She said that although her husband was always 'good' to her, sex always hurt and she never enjoyed it. She saw sex as an obligation, her marital duty.

'Last week, a new lady doctor came to our surgery and she came out to visit me. I told her about my womb – the first person I have ever told – and she put something up inside me. I've been walking round with a smile on my face all week: do you think it's a sin?'

As we discussed this further, it became clear that Evelyn was having multiple orgasms associated with a newly fitted vaginal ring pessary. The bigger picture was that she had never had an orgasm before and felt guilty at the sense of dishonouring her husband's memory, as 'this thing is giving me better feelings than the old man ever did!' She was tempted to have it taken out – until I recommended she keep it and enjoy it!

(At the time of this visit, I was a registered nurse and Evelyn's local Catholic priest.)

The trouble with women...

The French philosopher Michel Foucault (1984) once asked poignantly 'why we burden ourselves today with so much guilt for having once made sex a sin'. Various mental health fields of practice, across times and peoples, show how women have frequently been dogged by negative assumptions and treatment based solely on gender and/or sexual identity. Women are often portrayed as 'other' to men, and men usually come out on top (no pun intended). Problems based on gender and sexuality are even more noticeable when a woman 'deviates' from what is accepted in her culture or society, based on its usual (reproductive and heterosexual) rules and expectations, often called 'heteronormativity'.

Notions of what it is to be accepted as a girl or woman describe most females, because they comply with the gender roles and expectations placed on them. Others, however, find themselves stigmatised and excluded for reasons related to sex (the acts), sexuality or sexual health, which can affect their mental health. At the heart of the problem is not just that female gender, sexuality and certain sexual practices have been pathologised, but also that they have been subject to the scrutiny of the 'medical gaze' (Skolbekken, 2008). As Lafrance (2004) says, femininity is 'an acutely social phenomenon that must be worked at, achieved and continually renewed by its subject'.

Female strength and resilience

Evelyn's story relates to so many cultural messages for women, including female gender identity, sexuality, and marital and maternal roles and the associated expectations. All these aspects of life can affect a woman's overall health and well-being (Evans, 2013). Evelyn's story highlights a number of vulnerabilities or risk factors for poor mental health, but equally demonstrates her resilience throughout life.

The risk factors are the parental beatings (child abuse and domestic violence) and subsequent disfiguration Evelyn received as a young girl. Her legs were physically scarred: a discrediting mark or 'stigma' in the true sense of the word, which she chose to conceal from all but her husband. Her experiences also would also leave emotional scars, which are likely to have had a negative effect on her long-term mental health and self-perceived notions of being a woman: spending all her married life without experiencing the pleasures of sex and intimate union, enduring the chronic pain of a prolapsed womb, and having only one child (at a time when having more was the norm). The fact that she later felt guilty about the joys of sex, especially the pleasure given to her by an inanimate object, highlights what Foucault (1984) said about how easy it is for society to pathologise sex, to turn it into a scientific knowledge, which he called the *scientia sexualis*. Foucault referred to the other side of that coin as the *ars erotica* – the art of sex.

Implications for mental and sexual health: personal well-being

Evelyn's story relates to sexual roles and expectations placed on females from childhood into old age, in ways that have a negative impact on their holistic health and well-being. Evelyn experienced having an aspect of herself disregarded or stigmatised by others. The spirit of the Royal College of Nursing's (2011) guidance implies that such disregard is inhumane and tantamount to neglect or abuse in itself.

In relation to a person's sexuality or sexual being, many individuals 'suffer in silence'. They conceal stigmatising conditions, hiding them out of sight of others. This concealability has its own course; people have to work hard at constantly covering up that which they consider to be discrediting: with make-up, haircut or, in Evelyn's case, by wearing trousers. In Evelyn's case, there is also the potential to look back on a whole life with regrets; existential sadness that taps into depression. The depression can then have a knock-on effect in regard to her experiences of gender ('being a woman'), her relationships and her (lack of) sexual fulfilment.

Tips for family and friends

- Mental health and sexual – and for many, reproductive – well-being can be intricately linked with each other, affecting an individual's healthy love of themselves, and their capacity for relationships with others which extends over the life-course.

- Multiple stigmas, negative judgements and discriminations – including those from family members – are often attached to poor mental/sexual health and can be detrimental and destructive to holistic, personal well-being.
- Supporting and helping to build personal mental resilience can empower individuals to deal with sexual and reproductive health challenges they may face in life – including stigma and abuse – in ways which are positively enriching and constructive of a victim, through survivor, to thriver strategy.

References and further reading

Coulter-Thompson E (2016) Queering healthy sexuality. In *Queering Sexual Violence* (ed J Patterson). Riverdale Avenue Books.

Evans DT (2001) The stigma of sexuality: concealability and course. In *Stigma and Social Exclusion in Health Care* (eds T Mason, C Carlisle, C Watkins, *et al*). Routledge.

Evans DT (2013) Promoting sexual health and wellbeing: the role of the nurse. *Nursing Standard*, **28**, 51–58.

Farrell M, Corrin K (2001) The stigma of congenital abnormalities. In *Stigma and Social Exclusion in Health Care* (eds T Mason, C Carlisle, C Watkins, *et al*). Routledge.

Foucault M (1984) *The History of Sexuality: An Introduction*. Penguin Books.

Goffman E (1990) *Stigma: Notes on the Management of Spoiled Identity*. Penguin.

Lafrance M (2004) Femininity. In *Sexuality – The Essential Glossary* (ed J Eadie), p. 68. Arnold.

Royal College of Nursing (2011) *Older People in Care Homes: Sex, Sexuality and Intimate Relationships: An RCN Discussion and Guidance Document for the Nursing Workforce*. Royal College of Nursing.

Skolbekken JA (2008) Unlimited medicalization? Risk and the pathologization of normality. In *Health, Risk and Vulnerability* (eds A Petersen, I Wilkinson). Routledge.

Growing up female

Margot Waddell

'It is the hour of the stranger. Let the stranger now enter the soul.'
– D. H. Lawrence (1923)

It is over 90 years since D. H. Lawrence gave this eloquent evocation of the ordinary, yet extraordinary, impact of puberty on the personality and the ensuing course of adolescence. Yet adolescence remains the 'hour of the stranger', when the personality painfully develops into its adult self. Lawrence does not make gender distinctions, but there are significant differences between growing up female and growing up male. Below are some comments from girls attending a specialist adolescent clinic.

- 'I cannot bear mental pain.'
  A 17-year-old, whose left arm, covered with scratches and scars, told a desperate story, physical evidence of her inner psychological pain that she needed to inscribe on her own body in an attempt to get rid of inner, unbearable tension.
- 'I feel depressed and unlikeable. Basically, I hate my looks. I'm fat and ugly. I don't smile anymore – only when I puff or get drunk.'
  A 14-year-old with anorexia.
- 'I didn't feel wanted at home. I was always rowing with my mum and her new boyfriend. I suppose I just wanted someone to love me unconditionally – someone I could love too.'
  A pregnant 15-year-old.
- 'I wake up in a panic most nights. The exam pressure is impossible. I just want to cry all the time. It's hopeless.'
  An 18-year-old.

Each of these statements is a powerful expression of the intensities of adolescent pain and confusion, and of the often unstoppable urge to act, or act out – that is, to attempt to manage internal conflict by action, rather than by thinking or feeling. Girls tend to act against themselves, as a result of intellectual pressure, depression, poor body image, lack of self-esteem and separation anxiety (this last taking the form of a fear of rejection). The statements describe responses to unmanageable states of mind, and the problems they describe will be familiar to many.

What happens in the mind (the internal world) cannot be separated from what happens in the body and external world. Freud (1933) suggested strong links between adolescent states of mind and the nature of early psychological development:

> 'If we throw a crystal to the floor, it breaks; but not into haphazard pieces. It comes apart along its lines of cleavage into fragments whose boundaries, though they were invisible, were predetermined by the crystal's structure.' (p. 59)

These vulnerabilities and weaknesses relate to early life experiences: the mother or carer's personality, the care the individual received;, and also the baby's own personality: what she tried to communicate, the intensity with which she did so and her capacity to arouse responsiveness in her carer (see Chapter 11). The relationship between the ability of the parent to hold everything together, and the manner and intensity within which a girl can communicate her needs, is especially important during the turbulent transition into being a teenager. The adolescent girl is adapting to a new, sexual body with breasts and pubic hair, a changing body shape and the onset of menstruation, alongside increased sexual and aggressive drives. In addition, puberty is beginning at an ever-younger age.

Emotional changes

These changes are related to the individual girl's biology and sexuality. Psychologically, they are likely to be accompanied by swiftly fluctuating states of mind as the girl struggles to discover and establish a new position in relation to the family and the outside world. Anxieties are often intense, especially around gender identity, masturbation and sexual experimentation.

In the face of these changes, it is understandable that the adolescent girl might mimic more primitive, infantile emotional states. Her emotional state is often characterised by extreme feelings, mood swings and the tendency either to idealise or to put down herself and others. Anxiety about the self often takes precedence over concern for others. Disregard for parental values is a characteristic rite of passage and, in the attempt to establish an independent identity, this can sometimes involve feelings of excessive rejection. Such disregard may stir up a sense of emptiness and guilt, or even fears of loss, in the adolescent girl. This can fuel an intense need for reassurance, often of a very childlike kind, and sometimes this is played out sexually.

In addition to these internal pressures there are the ordinary, very hard, psychosocial tasks of adolescence, such as separating from parents, taking exams and deciding on a future career. Teenagers have huge doubts about their ability to manage separation, loss and independence. They often feel disillusioned with life in and beyond the family, mourn their lost childhood and miss their earlier relationships. The actual psychosocial and psychosexual tasks an adolescent will undertake differ considerably from early to late adolescence, from culture to culture and from person to person.

Girls and relationships

There is a broad consensus that girls find familial, friendship and sexual relationships to be more stressful than do boys. Girls more often turn difficulties inwards, becoming depressed, preoccupied with body image or hypochondria, dissatisfied and self-blaming. For example, the onset of anorexia is often linked not only to puberty-related changes and sexual fears, but also to exams and peer-group pressure. Any failure is taken as a personal failing.

Group identity can be constructive, but it can also be anti-developmental in the extreme. There has been an emergence of girl groups, a 'ladette' culture, and gangs of aggressive teenage girls. These girls express their own emotional fragility through an especially group-oriented and often bullying assertiveness, with out-of-control drinking, sexual predatoriness and shrill, mindless, often intimidating behaviour, which may be a way of coping with fears of hopelessness.

Girls and their families

A key aspect of the separation process is that adolescents are deeply ambivalent about what they do, and do not, want their parents to know about. Similarly, they often feel conflict as to which world they want to inhabit at any one time – the home or the peer group. Therefore, adults/parents may not know as much about adolescent behaviour as they think, especially when it comes to sex and substance use.

The clash between family values and peer pressures should not be underestimated. The peer group, especially in early adolescence, can take on almost tribal significance, establishing its own norms. The peer group can support the growing personality or, if too gang-like, can dangerously subvert it. The group can be alarmingly addicted to impulsivity and mindlessness, especially in relation to drugs, alcohol and sexual promiscuity. Within a peer group, girls can feel immense pressure to conform to its norms, even if they are at odds with what the individual girl would personally prefer.

Sexuality and teenage pregnancy

The wider availability of contraceptives has had a dramatic effect on adolescent girls. Sexual norms, too, are swiftly changing. The number of young people having sex before 16 years of age has steadily risen over the years, with high rates of unprotected sex and a clear link between parental divorce and early sexual activity (Jónsson et al, 2000).

For adolescents who lack solid parenting, the 'pseudo-solution' might take the form of sexual risk-taking. A teenage mother may identify as an idealised version of her own disadvantaged mother or, equally, she may identify with the baby, seen as an object of total maternal care. Almost every teenager who 'chooses' to get pregnant will talk in terms of a desire for unconditional love, both for and from the baby. Sadly, the harsh reality of caring for a baby with immature emotional (and financial) resources seldom lives up to this imagined ideal.

In the UK, readily available and confidential contraception for teenagers is finaly starting to reduce pregnancy rates, but the UK has more teenage mothers than any other western

European country, despite a high number of teenage abortions. Individual responsibility, for which the seeds are sown in the earliest years, is key and might prevent anxieties of the sort that lead to early sexual activity. Some sociologists think a decline in the conventional family structure in the UK, in contrast to other parts of Europe, is an important factor.

Teenage pregnancy can be a form of acting-out by a girl who has unmet emotional needs, and who harbours the delusion that a baby could be the way to meet them.

Body image

In the adolescent girl's world, the body so often becomes the focus of problems. As with young women with an eating disorder or who self-harm, the body can be the site of a battle royal that has to be fought, usually with parents (especially the mother – to achieve a sense of separateness and of identity) that is, by the girl's having achieved a sense of her own body and her own mind.

Conclusions

The psychoanalyst Irma Brenman Pick (1988) pointed out that,

> '[the] powerful forces and persuasive defences of adolescence may disturb or interfere with further growth; [but] they are also forces which make for the charm, vitality, enthusiasm and development of adolescents'.

The 'hour of the stranger' will eventually yield to the emergence of a grown-up self, drawing on the trials and tribulations of the teenage years as part of the ever-developing personality.

References and further reading

Brenman Pick I (1988) Adolescence: its impact on patient and analyst. *International Review of Psychoanalysis*, **15**, 187–194.

Freud S (1933) The dissection of the psychical personality. Reprinted (1953–1974) in the *Standard Edtion of the Complete Psychological Works of Sigmund Freud* (trans. & ed. J Strachey), vol. 22. Hogarth Press.

Jónsson FH, Njardvik U, Olafsdóttir G, *et al* (2000) Parental divorce: long-term effects on mental health, family relations and adult sexual behavior. *Scandinavian Journal of Psychology*, **41**, 101–105.

Lawrence DH (1923) Fantasia of the unconscious. Reprinted (2006) in *Fantasia of the Unconscious and Psychoanalysis and the Unconscious*. Dover Publications.

Part II.
Women and society

Poverty, exclusion, debt and women

Jed Boardman

The financial circumstances of the general populations have changed in the past few decades in the UK. Poverty and deprivation have disproportionate effects on people with mental health problems and on women in particular.

Poverty in the UK today

During the 20th century, huge improvements were seen in people's quality of life in the UK. Overall, standards of living, health, education and housing are better now than ever before. However, there were some significant changes in the later part of the century that are particularly relevant to women and women's lives.

From 1980 onwards, income inequality – the gap between rich and poor – dramatically increased. In the UK today, we seldom see absolute poverty, but there has been an increase in the numbers of people experiencing relative poverty (measured as an income of 60% or less of the median household income of that year): from 7 million people in 1979 to 13.8 million in 1997. In 2014, 13.5 million people, including 3.9 million children, were living in poor households (Joseph Rowntree Foundation, 2016; Tinson *et al*, 2016).

Despite some improvements in the 2000s, the situation has changed again since the 2008 recession. Although the UK has seen less unemployment than in previous recessions, wages have been stagnant and pay has fallen relative to prices. Now, having a job is no guarantee against being in poverty: of the 13.5 million UK households in poverty in 2014/2015, 7.4 million were families in which someone worked (Joseph Rowntree Foundation, 2016; Tinson *et al*, 2016).

Government targets set in 2010 to reduce the level of child poverty to 10% in 2020/2021 are unlikely to be met, and the predicted level of child poverty at that time is 24%. Housing costs have increased, there has been a rise in zero-hours contracts and job instability, and more people are underemployed. In 2012, 4.8 million people earned less than the living wage. More people are in debt, payday lenders charge high rates of interest, and there has been an increase in people using food banks. The pressure being applied to the poorest members of society has not been as great since before 1945, and attitudes towards the poor have hardened in recent years. The government's austerity measures have particularly hit the resources of health and social services.

Women with the added burden of a mental health problem face an even more challenging financial landscape. Since the recession, the unemployment rate for people with mental illness has risen higher than for people without mental illness. In addition, the changes in welfare provision have hit women with mental illness particularly hard. They face the brunt of the public sector cuts.

Social exclusion and disadvantage in women with mental illness

Having a mental illness means a woman is less likely to be able to participate in key areas of economic, social and political life, and that she is likely to be socially excluded. This applies particularly to those with severe and enduring mental health problems, such as schizophrenia and intellectual disability. Women with these conditions often lack material resources and have low incomes. They are commonly unemployed, having missed out on education, qualifications and training. They are likely to be isolated and excluded from social relationships, neighbours and the wider community. Disadvantages such as these can be both a cause and a consequence of having a mental illness.

Gender and mental illnesses

Overall, women and men have similar rates of diagnosed psychiatric disorders. However, when we look at the kinds of problems women experience, clear gender differences emerge. These differences are important in determining the needs of affected women and in delivering services better tailored to meet these needs.

From adolescence onwards, girls and women have higher rates of anxiety, depression, trauma-related disorders (such as post-traumatic stress disorder), eating disorders and somatoform disorders than boys and men.

Gender differences in the rates of these common mental disorders are likely to relate to social factors specific to women across the world:

- gender-based violence (e.g. domestic and sexual violence and abuse)
- socioeconomic disadvantage (e.g. poverty, hunger, malnutrition)
- low incomes and income inequality
- low social status
- responsibility for caring for others.

Feminisation of poverty

Globally, poverty is a destroyer of human lives for which many women shoulder the burden. This is clearly a matter of social justice and human rights, but reducing poverty also makes economic sense: it means more people can contribute to the economic good. Many studies have shown that poverty impairs child development and life chances (Wilkinson & Pickett, 2009; Boardman et al, 2010; Bennett & Daly, 2014).

A disproportionate number of the world's poor are women. Overall, 6 out of 10 of the world's poorest people are women. There are around 1.2 billion people in the world who live on less than $1.25 per day. More than 1 in 5 children in low-income countries live in absolute poverty and are vulnerable to malnutrition.

In the UK, poverty means lacking the material resources to meet an individual's minimum needs. For women in the UK, it is unlikely that resources are shared equally in low-income families, as a woman can get less than her fair share when children's needs are prioritised. Women are more likely to be single parents (especially young single parents) and to be carers of dependent relatives. Households with a disabled person are more likely to be poor than those without; a quarter of all UK families that include a disabled person are in poverty.

Families with children face the most difficulty in keeping up minimum income standards, a situation that is particularly difficult for lone parents. In the UK today, 40% of lone-parent families have a low income. Finding ways of affording extra costs when needed is particularly difficult for lone parents, who often have to do without essentials. Lone parents face the trap of needing adequate childcare to allow them to earn a wage, but childcare costs have risen disproportionately, critically disadvantaging women.

The gender gap: employment and pay

Gender inequality is manifest in many ways worldwide. The World Economic Forum has reported on the gender gap in over 120 countries since 2006. It focuses on health, educational attainment, workforce participation and political empowerment to calculate a Global Gender Gap Index. No country has closed the gender gap on employment or political participation, but 25 have closed it on education and 35 on health and survival. The five Nordic countries (Denmark, Norway, Sweden, Finland and Iceland) hold the top places and Yemen has the lowest ranking. The UK is in 26th place (World Economic Forum, 2014).

The UK's relatively poor ranking was in part the result of falling scores on employment: men have benefited more than women in this area during the recent recession. Nevertheless, there have been considerable changes in women's employment over the past 50 years, with current rates of female employment at around 67% (Office for National Statistics, 2013). However, significant gender gaps remain.

- Women are more likely to work part-time (three times as many women are in part-time work).
- Women have consistently lower employment rates over 22 years of age.
- Women's unemployment has risen over recent years and is now at a 25-year high.
- Women in full-time employment earn 15% less than men.
- Men make up the majority of workers in the top 10% of earners.

- The gender pay gap is greater in the private sector than the public sector.

The UK's progress in women's employment has faltered since the 2008 recession. In 2014, the UK ranked 16th out of 31 countries in the Women in Work Index (PwC, 2016). This poor ranking is attributed to above-average pay inequality and few full-time job opportunities.

Debt

Worldwide, 75% of people attempting to get loans cannot do so because they have unpaid or insecure jobs and do not own property. In the UK, there has been a significant increase in individual debt since 2008. In 2014, almost 1.4 million families (with 2.4 million children) are in 'problem debt'. In a separate study, two-thirds of the 8.8 million people in the UK very seriously in debt were women.

Mental illness can be both a consequence and cause of debt. Irresponsible practices of financial services can make individual debt worse. Those with mental health problems are particularly vulnerable to financial exploitation: compared with the general population, they are three times as likely to be in debt, and twice as likely to have problems managing their money. The consequences of debt can be devastating, creating a debt spiral that can lead to the eventual loss of important resources such as the home.

Inequality and generational effects of deprivation

Poverty and income inequality are harmful to individuals and society. Lack of material necessities is a direct cause of poor mental and physical health worldwide. Even in economically developed nations, income inequality is associated with poorer scores on measures of health (e.g. life expectancy, infant mortality, drug misuse, mental illness, obesity), social relations (e.g. trust, involvement in community life, homicide, imprisonment) and human capital (e.g. child well-being, social mobility, teenage pregnancies). Overall, more equal nations do better; Japan and the Nordic countries perform better than the UK. The harm seems to be related to 'status anxiety' – our sense of relative superiority and inferiority and worries about how others see and judge us. It may be possible to improve the quality of human life by reducing income differences.

Poverty and deprivation are dynamic. The effects can be time limited, but often they affect people over their entire lives and can affect subsequent generations. There are historical cycles of social disadvantage, whereby early life experiences (e.g. family disruption, educational disadvantage, poverty) contribute to poor social outcomes (e.g. mental illness), which then contribute to further disadvantage in the future. Children born into poor and disadvantaged families have poorer life outcomes than those born into better-off homes. Women and girls are especially vulnerable. Although mental health professionals have begun to acknowledge the effects of violence on women's lives and on their mental health, and to develop societal and service responses to these, we have yet to acknowledge the effects of poverty and deprivation in the same way.

Useful resources

Debt

Mind: Money and Mental Health
www.mind.org.uk/information-support/tips-for-everyday-living-money-and-mental-health

Rethink: How to Deal With Debt
www.rethink.org/living-with-mental-illness/money-issues-benefits-employment/debt-and-money-management

Gender gap

Fawcett Society
www.fawcettsociety.org.uk

Income inequality

The Equality Trust
www.equalitytrust.org.uk

Poverty

Joseph Rowntree Foundation
www.jrf.org.uk

United Nations Development Programme Human Development Reports
http://hdr.undp.org/en

References and further reading

Bennett F, Daly M (2014) *Poverty through a Gender Lens: Evidence and Policy Review on Gender and Poverty*. University of Oxford.

Boardman J, Currie A, Killaspy H, *et al* (2010) *Social Inclusion and Mental Health*. RCPsych Publications.

Joseph Rowntree Foundation (2016) *UK Poverty: Causes, Costs and Solutions*. JRF.

Office for National Statistics (2013) *Women in the Labour Market*. ONS.

PwC (2016) *Women in Work Index*. PwC (http://www.pwc.co.uk/economic-services/assets/PwC-Women-in-Work-2016-FINAL-3.pdf).

Tinson A, Ayrton C, Barker K, *et al* (2016) *Monitoring Poverty and Social Exclusion 2016*. Joseph Rowntree Foundation.

Wilkinson RG, Pickett, K (2009) *The Spirit Level: Why More Equal Societies Almost Always Do Better*. Allen Lane.

World Economic Forum (2014) *The Global Gender Gap Report, 2014*. WEF.

Arranged marriage

Chetna Kang

Meeting someone whom we love and who loves us back is something most people hope will happen to them some day. Many would like that relationship to develop into a lifetime commitment/marriage and raising a family together. Marriage can bring with it many relationships that can be supportive and enrich our lives. It is no wonder, then, that so much emphasis is put on meeting the right person and that there are now so many ways that we can meet that person, from online dating to culture-specific speed dating. Some people, however, have arranged marriages.

Arranged marriage: a positive experience

The concept of arranged marriage is something that the British population has now become more familiar with, owing to the variety of ethnicities of the people who live in the UK. Arranged marriages are common in, but not exclusive to, Eastern and Middle Eastern cultures. Marriage is seen as a way to make a positive contribution to society and as an opportunity for spiritual growth.

Much is done to ensure the two people are suited to each other, so that they will be able to honour their vow of marriage for the rest of their lives. However, the approach to arranged marriage varies considerably between different faiths and cultures, and even within a single culture it is influenced by education.

At one end of the spectrum, there are families where the parents and relatives act as an introductory agency and will do much of the checking and vetting that modern dating agencies do to ensure potential partners have the highest chance possible of being a good match. Add to that the fact that your family knows you better than most; this is becoming an increasingly popular choice among British Asians. Laila had her marriage arranged in this way.

Laila's story

Laila had been suffering with depression on and off since university. Her confidence had taken such a knock that even though men would take an interest in her, she felt that if they found out that she had depression, they would quickly lose interest and leave. That would leave her devastated and she did not want to take the risk. Her parents, however, were confident that she could meet someone who would accept her for who she was and with whom she could be honest. They and their close friends, at Laila's request, set about looking for men to meet in their community, who they felt would not reject her based on her mental health needs and who would also be suitable in terms of interests, personality and intellect.

After 2 years, Laila met the man who is now her husband. Through marriage, she found self-confidence, and when she does feel depressed, she tends to recover more quickly because of the love and support of her husband and their families. Laila says that marriage has been very positive for her and she couldn't have achieved it without the help of her parents.

Arranged marriage: a negative experience

Marriages do not have to be forced to have a negative impact on women's mental health. Some women with mental illness have reported that, in wanting to do something positive for their daughter, the parents had arranged a marriage; however, it was with someone who did not know about their illness. This left the women with the conflict of either hiding their illness or risking their partner leaving them once they are told. Anisha found herself in this situation.

Anisha's story

Anisha was diagnosed with schizophrenia when she was 19 years old. So long as she takes her medication, she lives a full and active life. As she entered her 30s, her parents started to worry about how she would manage once they were gone. Anisha was interested in getting married and her parents arranged a marriage with a man from Bangladesh. They met once and kept in touch over the phone. Anisha thought that her parents had told him about her schizophrenia and saw no reason not to marry him. When she found out they had not told him, it was too late. Anisha described the first year of her marriage as hell. She was in constant anxiety about being found out and this anxiety pushed her into a relapse. When her husband finally found out about her mental illness, he and his family felt let down and cheated. Anisha was too unwell to respond at the time; her husband is still in Bangladesh and they are trying to work things out.

Forced marriage

Laila's marriage was arranged at her request and was between two consenting adults who had shared important things about each other beforehand. However, not all arranged marriages meet the same criteria. They can vary in the degree of choice, consent and prior information about the other person. Although not common, this can be as extreme as the forced marriage of underage girls to significantly older men, often abroad. The impact of this on the emotional, psychological and physical health of the girls concerned can be devastating. If you or someone you know are in this situation, there are organisations that can help (www.gov.uk/forced-marriage).

Conclusions

Although Anisha and Laila's stories are in stark contrast, it is clear that when marriage takes place between two consenting adults who are well suited to each other, regardless of who introduced the two individuals, it can be a good start to a loving and happy partnership that is good for everyone's well-being.

Girls at risk

Trish O'Donnell

Bronagh's story

It all started when Bronagh was 13 or 14. A boy who used to go to her school added her as a contact on MSN after he left. Bronagh was surprised, as he hadn't liked her much and she hadn't really had anything to do with him. She thought maybe he wanted to catch up on news from his old school, so accepted his request. At first everything was fine, but then out of the blue he turned on her. He started saying nasty things about her and about her family, and it kept happening.

'He would make sectarian comments,' said Bronagh, 'calling me a nasty name for a Catholic rather than using my name. He'd say horrible things about how I looked – I'm a redhead, and he'd say that being ginger is a disability. He called me fat and ugly, and I really started to take it to heart. He said I should want to kill myself. Girls go on about their weight and worry about not being pretty as it is, and then I had this boy saying all these awful things, so I started to think it must be true. I started to believe that I was all the things he called me and my self-confidence was really low.

'I didn't talk to my family about it as the things he was saying about them were so hurtful too and I didn't even want to repeat them. He said my niece should never have been born, he said my parents should commit suicide for having a daughter like me, and he was abusive about my brother because he's gay.

'I know my family would have been supportive, but I just didn't want them to know what was happening. I spoke to some of my friends, and they were shocked. I think one of them challenged him over MSN about what he was doing, and he blamed me. I logged back on and he showed me these red marks on his neck over the webcam, and said that he'd tried to hang himself because of what I'd said about him. Then I started to feel like it was all my fault. I brought it to an end by permanently blocking him from my MSN account. I found out he was creeping Facebook to find out about me, so I changed my settings. Now I just wish I'd done it sooner – that I'd cut him off straight away and not let him get to me.'

Bronagh has used her experience to help others. After it happened to her, a friend experienced something similar. She was fighting with another girl on Facebook and it was getting really quite nasty.

'I asked her would she not talk to her mum,' said Bronagh, but she didn't want to, so I suggested contacting Childline. At first she didn't want to because she said she was afraid that whoever answered the phone would be judging her. I said if they did that they wouldn't be doing their job right, but I think I understand a bit better now why people maybe don't make the call. In the end she did use the online service and did the same thing as I did – blocking the person she'd had problems with. I would tell anyone who is experiencing anything like I did to take action and not let it go on. I've learned that if someone's behaviour isn't doing you any favours, then you need to block them straight away. I don't use MSN anymore, and on Facebook I only accept people as "friends" if I know, like and trust them in real life.' (Story included with permission from the National Society for the Prevention of Cruelty to Children (NSPCC).)

Being confident in who you are as a girl is a difficult challenge, even without any adverse experiences. For some girls growing up today, life can bring particular experiences that increase the risk to their mental health. For the parents of a girl, it is important to be aware of the challenges she faces, to talk with her about them, and to notice and respond sensitively to changes in behaviour. A change in behaviour is a symptom of something; it might be a normal developmental change, but it might be something else. There is a strong link between various types of abuse – particularly sexual abuse and bullying – and suicide attempts (Colquhoun, 2009).

Bullying and sexual bullying

Bullying is pervasive in our society. Many girls have been bullied or know someone who has been bullied. Bullying has the intention of causing harm or pain to someone, and can be physical or non-physical, face-to-face or digital.

Cruel comments or messages can be used to stalk, threaten, coerce and humiliate. Mobile phones and social networking are part of everyday life now, which means many girls who are the victims of bullying have little respite in our constantly connected world. Homes and bedrooms, which previously provided a private or safe space, are not safe from threats or taunts coming through a girl's phone or computer.

It is important not to underestimate the harm bullying can cause to girls and young women. It can make them feel scared, alone, ashamed and like they want to die. It can cause depression, self-loathing, self-harm and even suicide.

For girls and young women, bullying is frequently focused on their gender and their image of themselves as female. Girls are bombarded with perfect body images in the media, and being 'sexy' is a pressure that is virtually unavoidable. Sexual bullying can adversely affect girls, objectifying their bodies and appearance. Girls often experience:

- comments about body shape, size, clothes and looks (e.g. breast size, weight)
- being teased or put down because of their sex life (e.g. because they are a virgin)
- pressure to act in a sexual way or belittling of their sexuality (e.g. making fun of someone for being 'gay')
- name-calling, specific sexual words (e.g. 'slut' or 'bike')
- threats or jokes about rape
- spreading rumours or images about a girl's sexuality and sex life (e.g. graffiti, texts, posts on social network sites, tweets)
- unwanted touching (being touched in parts of the body that she does not want to be touched).

Which girls get bullied?

Bullying can happen to any girl. She has never 'brought it on herself' by any action or inaction. Shame can have a powerful effect on a young girl, causing her to keep the bullying to herself, and putting her at further risk.

There are some things that can be done so a girl or young woman is safer in specific situations, such as online. Like learning to cross the road, girls can be taught from an early age not to share anything (such as photos or private information) that they would not happily share with a stranger in the street, and not to accept friend requests from people they do not know; meeting them online does not mean that they know them.

What you should do if you find it happening to you or someone you know?

Don't keep it to yourself. Bullying thrives on shame and fear. Tell someone trustworthy, like a parent, carer or teacher. Schools will be able to help and tackle the problem at its source. Many schools have counsellors and some have peer-mentoring schemes to support pupils. There are all sorts of help available, and asking for it will make a difference.

As technology can be a weapon in the bully's armoury, it can also be a great help in combatting it. There are many websites and organisations that offer help, and some where young people can chat to others safely and securely and get advice about what to do (see the 'Useful resources' section at the end of this chapter).

If the impact of the bullying is severe and results in nightmares, panic attacks, phobias or self-harm, your general practitioner (GP) can help, perhaps by referring to the local child and adolescent mental health services (CAMHS). There might be a wait to see someone, so try the listed websites until a service becomes available.

Sexual abuse

For some girls, sexual abuse is a sad fact of their childhood. Sexual abuse has been linked to childhood and adult mental illness, including anxiety, depression and post-traumatic stress disorder.

Not every girl who experiences sexual abuse is affected to the same degree. Research findings vary, but suggest that 20–40% of women will show no serious ill-effects later in life. However, it makes growing girls more vulnerable to later mental health problems. Living with pain and trauma can lead to risky or harmful behaviours, delinquency, drug and alcohol misuse and dependency and other forms of self-harm. Strong self-esteem, self-reliance and positive coping strategies can help limit the effects of abuse. So can support from adults known to the child, or through school, religious groups or social clubs.

Getting help through supportive therapies can make a difference, as it can relieve aspects of distress and self-blame.

Being believed and supported by an adult who is important to the child is crucial. Talking therapies can support girls and young women who have been sexually abused. These include cognitive–behavioural therapy, psychodynamic psychotherapy and counselling, as well as more creative therapies, such as play therapy, art therapy or drama therapy.

Sexual abuse is a crime, and for services working with children there is a duty to report abuse. Many children do not disclose the abuse they experienced until they are adults, and some never do. Asking children if anything has happened to them can prompt them to tell – if not straight away, then at some future point.

Girls and young women value therapy that is accessible, non-judgemental and non-directive. They want space for humour, and value straight talking, trust and confidentiality. They like being listened to, but might not want to talk about the details of the abuse itself. Dealing with what it did to them – rather than what was done – is key.

Unfortunately, services for girls who have been sexually abused are not comprehensive and not available everywhere. Local CAMHS might only be available through GP referrals, and then only for symptoms of abuse, such as depression or self-harm, not the experience of abuse itself. Some areas have sexual assault referral centres (SARCs) for young people for the initial investigation period. Although SARCs are helpful in delivering care to victims of recent rape and serious sexual assault, they are not designed to offer long-term support. SARCs will, however, direct girls to longer-term therapeutic services, which are often provided by voluntary organisations, such as the NSPCC, Barnardo's or Childline (a service provided by the NSPCC). Practitioners who provide IAPT (improving access to psychological therapies) for children and young people might be available for further support.

Child sexual exploitation

Child sexual exploitation is a type of sexual abuse in which children are sexually exploited for money, power or status. Girls can be tricked into believing they are in a loving, consensual relationship. They might be invited to parties and given drugs and alcohol. They might also be groomed online or through their mobile phone. Some girls or young women are trafficked into or within the UK for the purpose of sexual exploitation. Sexual exploitation can also happen to girls in gangs.

How can you tell if a girl is being sexually exploited?

Running away or going missing can be an indicator that a girl is being targeted or already being sexually exploited. Those in residential care are three times more likely than other children to go missing.

Becoming trapped in an exploitative situation does not happen overnight. Early warning signs include the first going-missing episode, an older boyfriend who gives gifts or money, and being collected or dropped off by car if the driver keeps their distance and obscures their identity.

Drugs, alcohol and partying are often involved. Girls might be flattered and at first see it as a positive relationship, feeling 'loved'. It is characteristic of the exploitative relationship that the girls are groomed, and can see attempts to help them as actions against them. Talking to girls early on about making healthy choices can have some success, so education and early identification of risk are crucial.

Girls in care

Care can provide a safe and supportive environment for children and young people who have suffered harm, but children and young people generally find themselves in care because of adverse life experiences, such as abuse and neglect. Research has found that 45% of children in care have a diagnosable mental health condition (Meltzer *et al*, 2003; Ford *et al*, 2007). Overall, being in care means increased vulnerability, compared with other children.

There are over 30000 girls up to the age of 18 in care (Department for Education, 2013). It is difficult to know whether their increased vulnerability is caused by experiences prior to coming into care, or experiences while in care, but we do know that these girls need support to help them overcome these negative experiences.

It is vitally important that mental illness in girls in care is detected and treated. Since 2008, local authorities must monitor the emotional well-being of all looked after children via a questionnaire. This is a useful tool to quickly and easily assess any basic difficulties and to understand why problem behaviours have developed.

The positive aspects of ordinary care for looked after girls should not be underestimated, and good care, along with targeted help, can help in improving their mental health and well-being. These, along with involving girls and their families in consensus decision-making, are important in the long term (Luke *et al*, 2014).

Running away or going missing

Running away, or going missing, is a symptom of some form of distress. Girls are telling us something with this behaviour. Common reasons for running away include:

- family arguments
- family violence
- physical abuse
- sexual abuse
- problems at school
- pregnancy
- forced marriage
- running away from care
- neglect (not looked after properly at home)
- a stressful situation (e.g. the death of someone loved)
- problems with drugs or alcohol.

Going missing from home or school can leave any young person vulnerable, but girls are more likely to fall victim to sexual exploitation.

Gangs and girls

Girls in gangs are susceptible to sexual violence and exploitation. In a gang environment, this usually happens between young people who know each other, and it does not usually involve strangers in the wider community.

When young women are harmed through gang activity, it is rarely reported and so they rarely get help. Some of the reasons are fear of being punished, fear of it happening again with increased violence, and mistrust of services. Living in a negative environment or being surrounded by people who behave in a certain way can influence the way you see the world, and girls can even come to believe these things are normal. Being traumatised can lead them to bring others into the harmful situation. This behaviour can place other girls at risk, or can lead to further isolation, as other girls at school, for example, might stay away from them through fear.

If you are concerned about a girl you know, help and support are available through any of the organisations listed at the end of this chapter. Gangs and peers have a powerful influence on girls, but allegiance to a gang is (although hard) not impossible to overcome.

Useful resources

Abianda
www.abianda.com
Offers one-to-one/group work and employment opportunities for young women affected by gang association.

Barnardo's
www.barnardos.org.uk

Brook
www.brook.org.uk
0808 802 1234
Young people's sexual health and well-being.

Bullying UK
www.bullying.co.uk
Helpline: 0808 800 2222

Childline
www.childline.org.uk
Helpline: 0800 1111

Family Lives
www.familylives.org.uk
Helpline: 0808 800 2222
Support for parents and carers.

Girls in Gangs
http://girlsingangs.org
A student-led project that explores the issues around girls' involvement in gangs.

Losing Control: A Story about Sexual Exploitation
www.youtube.com/watch?v=XasNkfQ5AVM
NSPCC/Childline awareness-raising animation about young girls at risk of, or who have experienced, sexual exploitation.

Missing People
www.missingpeople.org.uk
Call or text: 116 000; email: 116000@missingpeople.org.uk

NSPCC
www.nspcc.org.uk
Helpline: 0808 800 5000
Provides support for adults who are worried about a child, advice for parents and carers, consultations with professionals who come into contact with children who have been abused or are at risk of abuse, and information about child protection.

Parents Against Child Sexual Exploitation (PACE)
http://paceuk.info

Safeguarding Children e-Academy
www.safeguardingchildrenea.co.uk
Online training aimed at equipping parents with the knowledge to protect their children against child sexual exploitation.

Safer London
www.saferlondon.org.uk
Supports young people through violence and exploitation.

Young Minds
www.youngminds.org.uk
Young people's mental health and well-being.

References and further reading

Colquhoun F (2009) *The Relationship Between Child Maltreatment, Sexual Abuse and Subsequent Suicide Attempts.* NSPCC.

Department for Education (2013) *Children Looked After in England (Including Adoption and Care Leavers) Year Ending 31 March 2013* (Statistical First Release, SFR 36/2013). DfE.

Ford T, Vostanis P, Meltzer H, *et al* (2007) Psychiatric disorder among British children looked after by local authorities: comparison with children living in private households. *British Journal of Psychiatry*, **190**, 319–325.

Luke N, Sinclair I, Woolgar M, *et al* (2014) *What Works in Preventing and Treating Poor Mental Health in Looked After Children?* NSPCC/Rees Centre.

Meltzer H, Corbin T, Gatward R, *et al* (2003) *The Mental Health of Young People Looked After by Local Authorities*. Office for National Statistics.

Domestic abuse

Roxane Agnew-Davies and Louise M. Howard

Kim's story

'My mother was always critical of me and my father left when I was a child. When John and I started going out, he was attentive and I felt I had found someone who cared for me at last. Looking back, his interested questions always turned into an interrogation about who had talked to or texted me, especially men. He became jealous and possessive, even though I was totally in love. Things got worse when I became pregnant. When I didn't feel like sex, he accused me of having an affair and called me a whore. Basically, I often had sex to keep the peace, even when I didn't feel well. I really didn't like oral sex, but as my belly got bigger, John insisted it was my job to give him pleasure. It really hurt a few times. I got more and more depressed, and John got angrier. I felt too ashamed to ask anyone about it, and I could never have told my mother something like that. Even if it was embarrassing, it was a relief when my midwife asked me if things were okay between me and my partner, and if we had any sexual problems during pregnancy. When I told her, she explained that it was sexual abuse if John did not take 'no' for an answer when I did not really want to have sex. She referred me to a Relate counsellor and that really helped. The counsellor saw us separately at first, and thinking about my rights and that I was not to blame really helped my self-confidence. I realised that I was a good person and I would rather be on my own than be put down or forced into things, by Mum or John. I left John for a while and that gave us both some breathing space. When Gemma was born, John promised that he would respect me and protect us both. It's good to have a family at last.'

What is domestic abuse?

Domestic abuse (or domestic violence) is a pattern of coercive and controlling behaviour by a partner or family member that can include physical violence, sexual violence, emotional/psychological abuse (such as humiliation) and financial exploitation.

Physical violence can range from minor assaults, such as a slap or a kick, to serious injuries that result in death. Sexual violence is any kind of sexual activity without consent – the willing agreement of someone to choose to have sex. It includes rape or penetration of the mouth, vagina or anus by a penis or an instrument such as a bottle or knife. Sexual assault is any kind of intentional sexual touching of somebody else without their consent. It is also child abuse if the person is under 16 years of age. Emotional abuse can be less obvious but can have a severe impact on mental and physical health. Women are much more likely to be victims of severe and repeated episodes of domestic abuse than men.

How common is domestic abuse?

Around 6% of all adults aged 16–59 have experienced domestic abuse in the past year (Office for National Statistics, 2016, 2017). Overall, 45% of women and 26% of men experience at least one incident of interpersonal violence in their lifetime (Walby & Allen, 2004); however, when there were more than four incidents (i.e. a pattern of ongoing abuse), 89% of the victims were women.

Men are far more likely to commit domestic abuse than women – in the year ending March 2016, 92% of defendants in domestic abuse prosecutions were male (Office of National Statistics, 2016). However, one survey found that a quarter of all gay and bisexual women have experienced violence within a relationship, and in two-thirds of these cases the perpetrator was female (Hunt & Fish, 2008).

What increases vulnerability?

Seeing domestic abuse or being abused as a child is associated with experiencing domestic abuse as an adult, but domestic abuse can happen to any woman. Some women are more vulnerable if their families or friends ignore or collude with the abuse, for example, by refusing to believe them or by forcing them into marriage.

How does domestic abuse affect women?

All experiences of domestic abuse are traumatic. A woman's reaction will depend on a lot of things, like what happened, what support she has, whether someone has hurt her before, and her personal strengths and situation.

Most women re-live or think about what happened, have bad dreams or feel confused. It is natural to try to push away these upsetting thoughts and feelings, but they might pop up anyway. Women might feel numb and want to avoid certain people and places. It is normal to feel afraid, jumpy or on edge, and also to feel down and negative. Women might feel differently about relationships than they did before, be irritable and have angry outbursts. It can be harder to concentrate, to manage everyday life, to socialise or to look forward to the future. A woman's view of the abuser and perhaps of herself might change. It can be hard to make sense of a world that is not safe, when you did not have the power to stop the abuse and when others did not help. Sexual difficulties are common after rape.

Tips for women who have experienced domestic abuse

Safety comes first. If you are still at risk, talk to someone close to you or to a helpline about making a safety plan to protect you from future harm. Think of yourself as a customer in a shop; if you do not find what you need the first time you look or ask, you try somewhere else (Box 8.1).

Healing can include coming to terms with what happened and being able to move on. Here are some ideas to think about.

- The abuse was outside your control and not what you wanted.
- What was done to you does not define you as a person because it was not your free choice or your fault, and is only one part of your life.
- Bad things happen to good people: 20% of women experience sexual violence and 25% of women experience domestic abuse.
- Many women do get over domestic abuse in their own time and learn to cope in their own way.

Box 8.1 Support organisations

- Free national domestic abuse helpline: 0808 2000 247
  www.refuge.org.uk
  www.womensaid.org.uk
- Forced marriage: www.fco.gov.uk
- Lesbian support services:
  http://lgbtdaf.org/category/lgbt-services-a-z
- Rape crisis centres: 0808 802 9999 (England and Wales),
  08088 010302 (Scotland)
- Sexual assault referral centres:
  www.thesurvivorstrust.org/sarc
  www.thehavens.co.uk (London)
- The Survivors Trust lists local specialist services across the UK
  and Ireland and offers information for survivors
  www.thesurvivorstrust.org

- It takes time, and you might work through shock, grief,
  anger and strong feelings about yourself and other people,
  not just the abuser.
- Take care of your body (e.g. medical checks, healthy
  eating, relaxation and exercise).

Understanding your reactions can help. Traumatic memories
are uncomfortable. It can help to know that there are reasons
they keep coming back:

- as a means to learn how to keep safe in the future
- because you could not process your thoughts and feelings
  at the time, when you were in a state of shock.

These memories can lessen when you have developed a
safety plan, and feel sure that the past cannot happen again.

Writing down what you were thinking and feeling at the
time and how it affected you, or better still, talking to someone
about it, can help recovery. Trying to bury the memories might
feel easier in the short term, but they can spring back, a bit like
trying to push a coiled spring down. If you start using drink or
drugs to block things out, that will not be good for you in the
long run – drug and alcohol use can worsen existing mental
health problems or even bring on new ones.

Help is available

Independent sexual violence advisors (ISVAs) are women trained to support victims of sexual assault and independent domestic violence advocates (IDVAs) are people trained to support victims of domestic abuse. They assess risks, can help with safety planning, give support during legal proceedings and contact other agencies.

Sexual assault referral centres have trained staff who can provide information, medical help and counselling. Medical support includes emergency contraception and screening for infections. Centres can help women speak to the police, although they will not pressurise women into doing so if they are not ready.

Rape Crisis Centres provide specialised support, counselling and advocacy for women who have experienced any type of sexual violence at any time in their lives, whether recently or in the past. This might be as an individual or in a group, and includes information and active support. Having someone who listens and understands can help women make sense of what happened and speed recovery.

Mental health problems resulting from domestic abuse, such as chronic or complex post-traumatic stress disorder, can be successfully treated with cognitive–behavioural therapy (CBT) or eye movement desensitisation and re-processing (EMDR), usually over 9 to 12 sessions. Using different methods, both of these therapies help with the processing of thoughts or memories about the abuse without feeling afraid and the development of resources to cope better. See Box 8.1 for a list of support organisations.

Tips for family and friends

Hearing that someone you love has been a victim of domestic abuse is shocking and disturbing, especially if you also know the abuser.

- Remember that the person responsible for the abuse was the abuser, not the victim. Try to be non-judgemental about her reaction and do not dwell on what you might have done.

- If you are angry or upset about what happened, be clear that you are *not* angry at the victim, but recognise that she is frightened and hurt.
- Ask what she needs for support.
- Remind her of the qualities, characteristics or skills you respect and admire about her.
- The best sort of support will mean leaving the door open for her to talk as much or as little as she wants, when she is ready, and for as long as she needs.

Useful resource

Online e-learning course

Social Care Institute for Excellence
Sexual Reproductive and Mental Health
http://www.scie.org.uk/publications/elearning/sexualhealth/

References and further reading

Bass E, Davis L (1988) *The Courage to Heal*. Vermilion.

Foa EB, Rothbaum BO (1998) *Treating the Trauma of Rape: Cognitive–Behavioral Therapy for PTSD*. Guilford Press.

Gil E (1988) *Outgrowing the Pain*. Dell.

Gil E (1992) *Outgrowing the Pain Together*. Dell.

Herman JL (1998) *Trauma and Recovery: From Domestic Abuse to Political Terror*. Pandora.

Hunt R, Fish J (2008) *Prescription for Change: Lesbian and Bisexual Women's Health Check*. Stonewall.

Matsakis A (1998) *Trust After Trauma*. New Harbinger.

Office for National Statistics (2016) *Domestic Abuse in England and Wales: Year Ending March 2016*. ONS.

Office for National Statistics (2017) *Crime in England and Wales: Year Ending Sept 2016. Statistical Bulletin*. ONS.

Walby S, Allen J (2004) *Domestic Violence, Sexual Assault and Stalking: Findings from the British Crime Survey* (Home Office Research Study 276). Home Office Research, Development and Statistics Directorate.

Women and the criminal justice system

Annie Bartlett

Jo's story

Jo is 38 years old. She has three children. She has a long history of street drug use and has been in contact with community drug services for over 10 years. More recently, she has also drunk alcohol heavily. She has had some previous contact with the criminal justice system as a result of her sex work, but only one episode of imprisonment following a minor assault. She has now been arrested because she stabbed her male partner.

She was seen at court by mental health liaison workers, but the seriousness of her criminal charge meant that she was remanded into custody. When she arrived in prison, she was sent to the prison wing specialising in drug and alcohol detoxification. At the end of this she seemed depressed and was seen by the mental health team. They established that, for many years, she had suffered with voices; these were unpleasant and distressing and dated from her experience of sexual abuse in childhood. She had self-medicated with street drugs from an early age and now, sober for the first time in years, she wanted other ways to manage her problems. She began attending a group to help her manage her voices.

She discussed her feelings of loss about her two oldest children, who were in care. Her youngest child lived with her mother. She was also worried about her offence. Although she was intelligent, it became clear that she lacked confidence. Her partner had undermined her and was periodically physically violent to her. She had poor basic literacy. She had never held regular employment.

There are a lot of women like Jo who are in contact with the criminal justice system. Most of them are, in fact, not violent but, if they are, the consequences can be serious not only for them, but also for their children. To understand how typical Jo's story is, let's explore common experiences in the background of female offenders, the kinds of mental illness they have, what happens after someone is arrested and the services that are there to help them.

Numbers, conditions and problems

Women constitute about 5% of the total prison population in the UK and about 15% of those who are under the supervision of criminal justice services in the community. Serious violent offending by women is rare and only a tiny number of women commit sexual offences. The total number of murder convictions in 2011 in England and Wales was 343, of which 23 (7%) were of women. Serious criminal cases are considered by the Crown Court, where 1 in 10 sentenced cases have female defendants. Less serious cases are heard at magistrates' courts, where women account for closer to 1 in 3 of those sentenced (Ministry of Justice, 2012a).

Female offenders often come from troubled backgrounds. Half have been physically or sexually abused in childhood, and a third have spent time in the care system. A third have been expelled or permanently excluded from school, giving them little chance of stable employment in adult life.

Approximately 1 in 5 prisoners who are 18–20 years of age have children, versus 4% of the general population in that age group. The consequences of a mother's imprisonment for these children can include having to move house, being looked after by the extended family, or being taken into care (Ministry of Justice, 2012b).

Women in contact with the criminal justice system are more likely to have mental health problems than women who aren't (Singleton *et al*, 1998; O'Brien *et al*, 2003). These problems can include major mental illnesses that require contact with specialist psychiatric services, as well as the kind of problems usually dealt with by general practitioners (GPs).

Many of these women have drug and alcohol problems. These are costly in physical, psychological and social terms. There are physical consequences, such as blood-borne viruses, blood clots and accidents. Women might experience social adversity stemming from sex work and street homelessness linked to addictions.

Difficulties in childhood frequently contribute to adult personality problems. Female offenders can be emotionally volatile, have problems forming stable adult relationships and commonly self-harm (particularly in prison custody). This is in addition to having a tendency to ignore social norms and break the law. The degree to which women have these problems is evident from the fact that many women in prison have more than one psychiatric disorder. Lately, it has been thought important to think not only about female offenders' mental health problems, but about other stressors they experience, such as having no stable accommodation, being in debt and experiencing violence in their adult relationships.

Female and male offenders tend to commit different crimes and have different mental health problems (Hodgkins *et al*, 1996; Wessely, 1997), and there are also gender-specific explanations of women's crime and violence (Farrington & Painter, 2004; Corston, 2007; Gelsthorpe, 2007). Broadly, women are less likely than men to be violent, but proportionately more likely to be violent to family members (e.g. partners, children), and more likely than violent men to have specific mental disorders. Women convicted of homicide are more likely to have a mental illness than men (Simpson *et al*, 2004; Flynn *et al*, 2011).

Treatment

Women in contact with the criminal justice system might be diagnosed with mental illness that requires treatment and/ or diversion out of the criminal justice system into the health service. Opportunities for these women to get treatment can occur when they are arrested, in the magistrates' court, on remand in prison, when they are sentenced for criminal offences, and after they have received a prison sentence. This system relies on close working relationships between criminal justice agencies and healthcare staff.

Historically, services to intervene early, in a process that can last many months, have not been a well-funded part of healthcare. Multiple reports have made recommendations to improve liaison between the courts and health services to allow diversion (Corston, 2007; Bartlett *et al*, 2012).

Entry to prison means undergoing a comprehensive screen on arrival for urgent and important health problems, including whether they need detoxification from street drugs and alcohol. Detoxification can lead to further psychosocial work on a woman's addictions, as well as slow withdrawal after stabilisation on opiates or benzodiazepines.

Routes of care after arrest include:

- diversion from police cells or magistrates' courts into specialist community healthcare
- custody (on remand or after sentencing) with care provided by health agencies in prison
- psychiatric hospital admission from court (magistrate or Crown) or from prison
- community criminal justice sanction with contact with GP services, community drug teams or community-based mental health teams.

Women charged with serious offences will probably come to trial. Even if mental illness has contributed significantly to their offences, they are likely to be convicted prior to any hospital placement. The assessment of future risk will also be relevant; courts consider carefully the likelihood of serious harm to anyone in the future. Particular legal measures can be put into place to reduce this likelihood, even if the woman goes to hospital. In the case of a violent offence, if a woman goes to a psychiatric hospital, it will be to a secure unit. There, a range of psychological and pharmaceutical treatments will be available to them.

Most women have short stays in prison, with only a small percentage of women serving more than 12 months. Women with convictions for violence are more likely to receive longer sentences. A range of primary care, psychiatric and psychological services are available in prison, depending on need and circumstance. Trials of psychological interventions have mainly been undertaken in other jurisdictions (e.g. for trauma symptoms and substance misuse).

Sentence planning is led by HM Prison and Probation Service staff and can involve placement in particular prisons with specialised services. For example, HMP Low Newton is suitable for women who pose particularly high risks, by virtue of personality disorders, and HMP Foston Hall offers the CARE (Choices, Actions, Relationships, Emotions) programme for women serving long sentences. Health and social care staff should work closely with criminal justice staff to make sure that all the woman's needs are met.

After prison

Coming out of prison, women might gain assistance from criminal justice agencies and specialist care, either in the National Health Service (NHS) or the voluntary sector (e.g. Women in Prison). The intention is to help women settle back into community life and to improve their opportunities and quality of life. The reoffending rate after 1 year for women is 17.6% (compared with 27.0% for men; Ministry of Justice, 2012*a*).

Conclusions

The existing, imperfect system of care for women in contact with the criminal justice system is changing rapidly. Both the number and type of women's prisons, as well as the secure hospital system, were reviewed by the government (Robinson, 2012). There was a new emphasis on housing women in prisons in metropolitan areas to help them maintain family contact, and an attempt to reserve secure hospital care and imprisonment for the small number of women who pose a risk to others. Despite the closure of HMP Holloway in 2016 and the relocation of many London female prisoners to prisons in Surrey, this remains the government's intention. A strategy on women offenders is due to be released, and the current plan is to create five community prisons to improve rehabilitation chances for women like Jo (Ministry of Justice, 2016).

Tips for family and friends

- Prison and secure hospital visits need to be organised in advance, especially if they involve children. Information on visits and what to expect if someone you know is in prison is available from the Prison Reform Trust's website (www.prisonreformtrust.org.uk/ForPrisonersFamilies/Frequentlyaskedquestions).

- Leaving prison or hospital is a welcome but often difficult step, during which women need support. There are a range of organisations that can help with this, including Women in Prison (www.womeninprison.org.uk) and Wish (www.womenatwish.org.uk).

References and further reading

Bartlett A, Somers N, Reeves C, *et al* (2012) Women prisoners: an analysis of the process of hospital transfers. *Journal of Forensic Psychiatry and Psychology*, **23**, 538–353.

Corston J (2007) *A Review of Women with Particular Vulnerabilities in the Criminal Justice System*. Home Office.

Department of Health (2002) *Women's Mental Health: Into the Mainstream*. DoH (http://webarchive.nationalarchives.gov.uk/20050315021049/http://www.dh.gov.uk/assetRoot/04/07/54/87/04075487.pdf).

Farrington D, Painter K (2004) *Gender Differences in Risk Factors for Offending. Findings 196*. Home Office.

Flynn S, Abel KM, While D, *et al* (2011) Mental illness, gender and homicide: a population-based descriptive study. *Psychiatric Research*, **185**, 368–375.

Gelsthorpe L, Sharpe G, Roberts J (2007) *Provision for Women Offenders in the Community*. The Fawcett Society.

Harty M, Somers N, Bartlett A (2012) Women's secure hospital services: national bed numbers and distribution. *Journal of Forensic Psychiatry and Psychology*, **23**, 590–600.

Her Majesty's Chief Inspector of Prisons for England and Wales (2007) *The Mental Health of Prisoners: A Thematic Review of the Care and Support of Prisoners with Mental Health Needs*. HM Inspectorate of Prisons.

Hodgkins S, Mednick SA, Brennan PA, *et al* (1996) Mental disorder and crime: evidence from a Danish cohort. *Archives of General Psychiatry*, **53**, 489–496.

Ministry of Justice (2012a) *Statistics on Women and the Criminal Justice System 2011*. MoJ.

Ministry of Justice (2012b) *Prisoners' Childhood and Family Backgrounds: Ministry of Justice Research Series 4*. MoJ.

Ministry of Justice (2016) *Prison Safety and Reform*. MoJ.

O'Brien M, Mortimer N, Singleton N, *et al* (2003) Psychiatric morbidity among women prisoners in England and Wales. *International Review of Psychiatry*, **15**, 153–157.

Robinson C (2013) *Women's Custodial Estate Review*. National Offender Management Service.

Simpson AIF, McKenna B, Moskowitz A, *et al* (2004) Homicide and mental illness in New Zealand, 1970–2000. *British Journal of Psychiatry*, **185**, 394–398.

Singleton N, Meltzer H, Gatward R (1998) *Psychiatric morbidity among prisoners in England and Wales*. TSO (The Stationery Office).

Wessely S (1997) The epidemiology of crime, violence and schizophrenia. *British Journal of Psychiatry*, **170** (Suppl 32), s8–11.

Part III.
Women and their environment

Emotional well-being and staying well

Kamaldeep Bhui and Zenobia Nadirshaw

Women face many challenges in the course of their lives that are less common in men's lives or that women experience differently from men. Four areas in which women face particular challenges are work, caregiving, education and exercise.

Work

Most women have children and women are usually the main caregivers; 80–90% of single parents are women. The lack of joint parental leave and benefits in the UK may mean that the salary of the lower-earning partner in a couple is more likely to be sacrificed to maintain family income. This may mean women either return to work part time or, for some women, working and earning a living becomes less of a priority. Some women may also lose the sense of achievement that work can provide once they become mothers. If they return to work on a part-time basis, generally, they have less opportunity for advancing their careers than men. In some societies and cultures (including in the UK), women have restricted workplace roles and any attempt to break free of these is shunned or stigmatised.

Despite progress, women continue to be underrepresented in senior positions in business, education, and private and public institutions, and to occupy more lower paid and part-time positions. Some believe that 'voluntary' childcare responsibilities contribute to that, but others have argued that childcare is poorly valued and given less respect compared with workplace progression. As time out from the workplace costs women experience, promotions and salary raises, and because women are less likely than men to ask for salary raises and promotions, it is easy to see how this may create a 'feedback loop' that reinforces the expectation that women will be the ones to take time off work. Affordable childcare and safe environments in which women can raise children, with sufficient social support and personal health protection, are important elements in preventing the discrimination in the workplace associated with having children. Recent changes to maternity/parental leave (i.e. shared leave) are a good first step, but in themselves are not likely to be enough to challenge the societal assumption that women are the primary caregivers and should sacrifice their careers.

Caregiving

Most caregivers in the UK are women. Longstanding caregiving for a loved one with a chronic condition can cause emotional strain. However, the most well-known form of illness associated with the burden of caregiving for women follows childbirth (see Chapter 31). This is one of the most common risk periods for severe mental health problems in women, including psychosis and severe depression. At its most tragic, postnatal mental illness can result in suicide and infanticide. In some cultures, girl babies are not valued; strong traditions exist where male children hold greater value because of future potential in terms of wealth and work, and because of the costs of dowries for families. These sentiments may seem outdated, but to some extent such subcultures still exist, in the UK and globally, often in association with poverty, poor literacy and lack of education.

Women are more likely than men to be carers of children with intellectual disabilities. These children may often have severe behavioural and physical problems. One study compared Asian and White families that included members with intellectual disabilities where the mother was the main carer (Azmi *et al*, 1996). Mothers were overburdened from their caring role in combination with running the household and their 'duties' as a wife, mother and daughter-in-law. Particularly for Asian mothers, stress and predisposition to mental illness were very high. They seemed one step away from crisis and breakdown, for which they would need specialised services for depression and anxiety. The study also found that mothers had not received help from statutory services for their children because they were afraid that, if they approached social services, the children would be taken away and they would be accused of bad parenting. Mothers who are struggling even with developmentally well children report similar concerns. The emotional journey of becoming a parent and the emotional, financial and other demands of looking after children can become overwhelming if the parent's own experiences of being cared for include cruelty, punishment or even physical and sexual abuse. Single mothers face special challenges in that they may have less immediate social support, unless they are living with extended family or close to friends who are willing to help with childcare. Public mental health interventions aim to reduce risk factors and increase protective factors in the population at different stages in a woman's life.

Women are also more likely to act as carers to elderly and unwell relatives and spouses with chronic illness. Carers report high rates of mental health symptoms and poor quality of life. Women acting as carers report being isolated and lacking independence compared to men in the same family. As carers and parents, women can struggle, especially if they are on a low income, socially isolated or without a supportive family network. Fragmented social networks in urban settings can also place women at risk of isolation. Women who have experienced traumatic events earlier in their live may also experience difficulties regulating their emotions, which can reduce their ability to develop and sustain nurturing relationships. Managing health and lifestyle risk factors can become difficult in these circumstances. Women may turn to smoking, alcohol use, drug use and, when encountering mental health problems, self-harm and thoughts of suicide.

Education and attainment

In the UK overall, more girls attain GCSEs and A levels, and at higher grades than boys, which is likely to be because of differences between girls and boys in language and literacy skills, and the fact that girls perform better in English and other subjects which are literacy based. This isn't the case for maths or science subjects which rely less on literacy. Girls also work harder at school overall. However, social class can have an even greater effect than gender, especially for some groups, such as

African Caribbean boys. Focusing on boys' underachievement does not address the fact that large numbers of girls are also low attainers. A report from the UK Department for Education and Skills (2007) stated:

> 'Tackling the scale of these numbers is arguably of greater priority and importance to policy makers than the proportionate difference between boys' and girls' attainment. Additionally, the different subject choices made by boys and girls may be more marked and have greater longer-term outcomes in terms of subsequent career choices than attainment differences.' (p. 5)

In schools in the UK, there is also evidence that girls have educational benefit from single-sex classes, which may be because they tend, as a group, to be less disruptive. More recent figures also indicate that girls' educational achievements are not holding them back in applying for further education, although they tend not to achieve the highest levels of income compared with boys with the same level of educational achievements/potential.

From an international perspective, Malala Yousafzai, the young Pakistani girl shot through the head by extremists who did not wish girls to be educated, highlights the importance of education in reducing gender-based discrimination and inequality globally. Some of these prejudices against girls' education are very present in ethnic groups in the UK today. Malala's championing of the education of women is important: access to education is key for women to achieve greater autonomy and self-efficacy in their lives, and to derive the associated advantages of better health, better mental health and well-being. Some of the effects of higher educational achievement are likely to be economic: people with more education tend to earn more and this reduces mental health risks. For women, the effects of education on autonomy and social power may be additionally important, especially in some cultures. In the UK, African Caribbean women have far better mental health and have been far more socioeconomically successful than their male counterparts. Women may be more able to manage change than men. This might be particularly relevant for newer groups of migrant women coming into the UK. However, unlike the Windrush generation, many recent migrant women have experienced significant trauma (violence, rape, loss of loved ones and children) which is likely to add to the hardships of migration.

Exercise and physical health

In the UK, women remain at an advantage in longevity, but the gap is closing rapidly. For older generations of women, however, who are far more likely to outlive men, there is a greater likelihood of isolation and loneliness in old age. Women are, in general, better at maintaining social relationships than men, and social networks are important as a protective factor for physical and mental health. Nevertheless, women are as likely as men to suffer from chronic and life-threatening diseases, so it is important for women to take care in managing risk factors for heart disease, cancer and dementia (see Chapter 13).

By 35 years of age, women begin to lose their female hormones. This loss continues until menopause, which occurs on average around 50 years of age. Later, aged about 75, women lose further remaining oestrogen when their adrenal glands begin to lose functionality, at so called 'adrenopause'. Oestrogen gives women an advantage in heart disease and stroke risk over men generally, but in later life this advantage lessens. Exercise appears to help maintain women's advantage in cardiovascular health over men, especially if women begin to exercise regularly by middle age (see, for instance, NHS Choices (www.nhs.uk) for type and amount of regular exercise recommended). Overweight, smoking and alcohol may disadvantage women more than men, however. In women with mental illness, the negative effects on physical health of medications are more pronounced than for men, and this needs to be taken into account when considering treatment choices and dosing and duration of drugs.

Tips for women to protect their well-being

- Exercise is helpful in preventing heart disease and depressive illness.
- Exercise should be regular (150 min a week) from middle age.
- Eat a nutritionally balanced diet and limit the intake of high-calorie, high-fat foods.
- As women metabolise alcohol more slowly than men, and are likely to suffer more damage from excessive alcohol use, limiting alcohol intake is also important.

- Maintaining social contacts and engaging in activities is important for maintaining mental health, which in turn will improve mental and cognitive health.

References and further reading

Azmi S, Emerson E, Caine A, *et al* (1996) *Improving Services for Asian people with Learning Disabilities and Their Families*. Hester Adrian Research Centre/The Mental Health Foundation.

Department for Education and Skills (2007) *Gender and Education: The Evidence on Pupils in England*. DfES Publications.

Gender and Women's Mental Health, a report prepared by the World Health Organization, and their website (www.who.int/mental_health/ prevention/genderwomen/en/).

Promoting Mental Health 4 Life, a learning resource to help individuals and organisations improve mental health (mentalhealthforlife.org).

Resources on women and mental health produced by the Mental Health Foundation (www.mentalhealth.org.uk/a-to-z/w/women-and-mental-health).

Sensitive motherhood

Helen Minnis and Philip Wilson

Parenting: a natural instinct

Parental sensitivity is a natural instinct (Kringelbach *et al*, 2008). When any adult hears a baby cry, she or he will have an emotional reaction (although the emotional reaction might be stronger in women than in men; Sander *et al*, 2007). This natural instinct was demonstrated in a study in which adults were asked to look at images of infants and adults (not from their own family or group of friends) while a magnetic resonance imaging (MRI) scanner measured the blood flow in different parts of their brains. When the image was of a baby, there was a lot of activity in the frontal and temporal parts of the brain; these areas are involved in planning complex behaviours (Kringelbach *et al*, 2008). When the image was of an adult, there was no such activity.

The fact that parental sensitivity is so natural means that it does not require conscious effort. It is something we can literally do without thinking. A sensitive mother is getting on with her life, but has in-built 'antennae' that allow her to be ready for action if her child is in need. The best example of this is the play park, where you will often see two women engrossed in a conversation with each other on a park bench, while their young children are absorbed in play. These women are not ignoring their children: they each have an 'ear out' for trouble. If a scary dog came into the park, the children would abandon their play and run towards their mothers. The mothers (if sensitive) would immediately abandon their conversation, in mid-sentence if necessary, and hold out their arms for a hug and some soothing words. Only when the crisis is over, and the children are once more engrossed in play, will the conversation between the friends resume.

Things that can block sensitivity

So what might get in the way of a mother being sensitive to her child? Anything that preoccupies the mind enough to stop the antennae from working. If there is insufficient support from family/friends, or complicating factors, mothers may find it difficult to be sensitive (Kivijärvi *et al*, 2001; Ensink *et al*, 2016). This was beautifully expressed by a new mother who had an infected Caesarean scar and postnatal depression, both of which preoccupied her so that she could not focus attention on her children. As she said, 'Until you can tune into yourself, you can't tune into your children'. Any number of things can block parental sensitivity.

A woman might have had a bad parenting experience with her own mother or father. She might have been told, when hurt as a child, that 'big girls don't cry'. If, in addition, that same mother is stressed by debts, an unsatisfying relationship with her child's father and the way her own mother constantly undermines her, she may not have the capacity to be nurturing when her child seeks attention. From the child's perspective, when she reaches out to be picked up, she is likely to get a grumpy response or be ignored. Such a child will eventually learn not to approach her mother at times of distress, although she might also learn that naughtiness always gets attention. The result can be a situation where the child becomes more and more challenging, and the mother becomes even more stressed, tired and less sensitive.

Or a woman might be living with domestic violence. She might be able to enjoy tuning into her child for most of the day, but as the time of her abusive partner's arrival home nears, she starts to tune out from her child and worry about staying safe while he is around. This is very confusing for the child. Why is Mum sometimes there for me and sometimes not? Children in this situation sometimes 'turn up the volume' and become whiny and clingy in the hope of getting the tuned-in care that they want. A vicious circle develops where the mother becomes increasingly stressed and irritated with her increasingly whiny child, and the pair end up with less and less tuned-in time.

Another mother might be addicted to heroin. She may enjoy life with her child when she has enough of the drug she needs, but as withdrawal starts to kick in, she will become more and more preoccupied with getting her next fix and less and less tuned into her child.

Alternatively, a mother might have experienced abuse and neglect in her own childhood. Sometimes trauma in the early months and years of life can lead to poorly processed memories that can result in flashbacks to frightening past events (i.e. memories that come back and 'bite you' when you least expect it). When the child reaches out to be picked up, this mother might be catapulted into her own past and might 'zone out' for a few moments. This can be very frightening for the child, who might be uncertain about whether to approach or avoid her in times of stress, in case 'that strange thing happens to Mum'.

The sensitivity continuum

These examples may seem a little extreme. But studies increasingly show that the quality of parenting a mother has received from her own mother or father has an important effect on her ability to parent her own children. This may explain why the parenting sensitivity of quite healthy mothers varies naturally from low sensitivity to an infant's cries (or other non-verbal cues) to high sensitivity. Most of us fall somewhere in the middle, so we talk about there being a continuum, or range, of parenting sensitivity (Kok *et al*, 2015).

Effects of parenting on the child

Lack of parental sensitivity can have serious long-term consequences for a child, beyond simple behaviour problems. It is not only genes that determine a child's abilities: sensitive, consistent and engaged parenting is required for the healthy development of language skills, the ability to profit from education (e.g. the child's ability to pay attention) and the formation of good relationships with others. Lack of engaged parenting early in life is associated with a range of problems in brain development, as well as psychiatric disorders in childhood and later life.

Studies of the effects of extreme emotional neglect, as occurred famously in Romanian children's homes, provide graphic evidence of the smaller brains of these children compared with non-neglected children of similar ages (Mehta *et al*, 2009).

Being a sensitive mother can be a fun and, at times, relaxing experience. Children need freedom to explore and learn from the environment, all the time being assured that the mother (or other carer) they trust and rely on is close by. This means that a sensitive mother can spend at least some of her time getting on with adult tasks, having her antennae up in case the child wants or needs her attention.

By contrast, factors associated with inadequate parental sensitivity tend to worsen an already difficult situation, because they result in a frustrated child and an even more stressed mother. So, how can we release mothers and their children from the shackles of 'blocked' sensitivity?

Improving parental sensitivity

One powerful technology that can help is video feedback. There are now various techniques (e.g. video interactive guidance, Mellow Parenting) in which participants are invited to review, along with a therapist, short video clips of themselves playing or interacting in other ways with their children. The purpose of this is to help the parent pay attention to what happens in the interaction, and therefore get a better understanding of what the child might want out of the interaction, and of the child's current needs. When interactions are working well, the child usually leads the communication (which can be completely non-verbal and as simple as an enquiring or checking look) and the parent follows instinctively.

It is amazing that, even in the most stress-filled relationships, it is possible to find at least a moment when interaction has worked well – probably because this is instinctive and we really can't help it. Seeing those lovely moments of contact can be reassuring and encouraging for a parent who is having difficulties – a bit like that moment when we are learning to ride a bike and we experience the 'whee' feeling. This can turn around a vicious cycle and begin a virtuous one, where the mother becomes more and more confident that she really does have a natural instinct to parent and can begin to relax into her role. Fairly short programmes of intervention (just a few weeks) can be very effective in improving parental sensitivity (Bakermans-Kranenburg *et al*, 2003).

In some Scandinavian countries, when a mother goes to her general practitioner complaining that she is not getting on with her baby, it is seen as an emergency and the kind of help we have just described is prescribed straight away. This makes sense when we consider how important even the earliest experiences are to a child's long-term development. Parental sensitivity is a natural instinct that, for some parents, just needs some help to be released.

Tips for women who want to improve parental sensitivity

- Parenting is instinctive – there is no special technique to it, other than what comes naturally.
- Sensitive parenting is led by the child – so sensitive parents can get on with their lives and have an 'ear out' for when their child needs something or wants to communicate.
- If there are problems with parental sensitivity, it usually means that there is a block somewhere, for instance, because of stress or lack of support.
- It is important to address problems with sensitivity because parental sensitivity is crucial for healthy development of language, attention and relationship skills.
- Short programmes of therapy – especially those involving video, such as video interaction guidance – can have a powerful positive effect on sensitivity.

References and further reading

Bakermans-Kranenburg MJ, van IJzendoorn MH, Juffer F (2003) Less is more: meta-analyses of sensitivity and attachment interventions in early childhood. *Psychological Bulletin*, **129**, 195–215.

Ensink K, Normandin L, Plamondon A, *et al* (2016) Intergenerational pathways from reflective functioning to infant attachment through parenting. *Canadian Journal of Behavioural Science/Revue canadienne des sciences du comportement*, **48**, 9–18.

Kivijärvi M, Voeten MJM, Niemela P, *et al* (2001) Maternal sensitivity behavior and infant behavior in early interaction. *Infant Mental Health Journal*, **22**, 627– 640.

Kok R, Thijssen S, Bakermans-Kranenburg MJ, *et al* (2015) Normal variation in early parental sensitivity predicts child structural brain development. *Journal of the American Academy of Child and Adolescent Psychiatry*, **54**, 824–831.e1.

Kringelbach ML, Lehtonen A, Squire S, *et al* (2008) A specific and rapid neural signature for parental instinct. *PLoS ONE*, **3**, e1664.

Mehta MA, Golembo NI, Nosarti C, *et al* (2009) Amygdala, hippocampal and corpus callosum size following severe early institutional deprivation: The English and Romanian Adoptees Study Pilot. *Journal of Child Psychology and Psychiatry*, **50**, 943–951.

Sander K, Frome Y, Scheich H (2007) FMRI activations of amygdala, cingulate cortex, and auditory cortex by infant laughing and crying. *Human Brain Mapping*, **28**, 1007–1022.

Religion and spirituality

Julia Head

Sonia's story

Sonia had always been part of her faith community, which she found supportive at many times during her life. She attended worship on a regular basis, but more recently her weekly attendance had turned into a daily routine and she became distressed when other responsibilities in her life threatened to disrupt the frequency of her visits. Sonia's partner became increasingly concerned about this change in her lifestyle and contacted her general practitioner (GP), who suggested that Sonia might find it helpful to discuss this with a spiritual advisor. It emerged that Sonia was very anxious about her elderly mother, who had been diagnosed with a heart condition. When she was able to discuss this with the spiritual advisor, her anxiety lessened. She was appreciative of being able to speak about what was happening in her wider relationships in the light of her faith.

When people are unwell or experience some kind of distress, they usually search for an explanation for their condition, its cause and what might help their recovery. In addition to searching for physical explanations and treatments, they might focus more deeply on the meaning of what is happening in their lives as a whole.

Spirituality *v.* religion

Many people do not have a specific religion, but still refer to spiritual needs and resources, particularly at difficult times. For instance, they might say, 'I'm not a religious person, but I do think of myself as spiritual'. Spirituality and religion are integrally related, but there are important distinctions to be made.

Spirituality is concerned with the search for ultimate meaning, truth and orientation in life. There are many dimensions, and many individual expressions, of spirituality. Religion in its many forms – worship, ritual, prayer, social groupings and so on – is a more 'corporate' concept. Spirituality often expresses itself through religion, but it tends to be a more personal concept, concerned with meanings and essential values. It is often important to be able to see beyond what seems to be a 'religious' problem to discover the meanings that individuals attribute to their lives and challenges. Sonia's story is a good example of this, where the increasingly obsessive religious behaviour is secondary to (and could indicate) underlying spiritual/existential concerns.

The pros and cons of religious/spiritual belief

Much research has been carried out into the complex relationship between mental health and spirituality/religion, but substantially less attention has been given to the gender differences in this relationship. Women are more likely than men to hold religious beliefs (Trzebiatowska & Bruce, 2012). Does an individual's spiritual/religious belief and behaviour promote mental and emotional well-being and increased resilience to adversity? Or can it have more negative effects? The answers are likely to depend on a number of factors, such as the woman's health status, maturity and psychological insight.

Faith as a protective factor

Spirituality and religion can be protective factors in women's mental and emotional well-being. For some women, spirituality can provide a means of defence against everyday difficulties, responsibilities and conflicts or a way of managing anxieties about death or dealing with actual or imagined wrongdoing. Religious beliefs can also give a sense of control over the human condition, and alleviate feelings of powerlessness and helplessness. A woman's psychological defences are her way of coping with life's challenges.

Research on coping has shown that people's spiritual and religious lives provide positive support and comfort when stressful life situations threaten mental well-being (Koenig *et al*, 1998). Some research suggests that women in general, including trauma survivors, are more likely than men to have positive religious coping skills (Fallot & Heckman, 2005). Other research has found that higher levels of spirituality in older women increase resilience, which is needed for successful ageing (Vahia *et al*, 2011).

Feeling that one has a personal relationship with a deity can be a protective factor in mental health, reducing stress and heightening self-esteem. Religious belonging and faith/spirituality are protective factors against suicide. Ritual, especially worship and prayer, can help a woman feel in control of her life: the repetitive nature of rituals gives security at times of tension, instability and self-doubt. It can also promote group closeness, strength and the possibility of emotional/cathartic release (perhaps its most significant characteristic).

An additional protective factor is the social support that belonging to a faith community can bring (Reid-Arndt *et al*, 2011). Many people view their communities as the first port of call when they are unwell. This social support, which can enhance quality of life, can be understood in various ways. Local groups can aid a woman's socialisation process, a vital factor linked to recovery, if previous relationships and social supports have been lost. The group can also provide practical support (e.g. financial assistance, food).

Health education is often encouraged through local faith groups and, in communities where appropriate and sensitive responses are made to mental illness, women can draw on the support of others in their attempts to cope with their problems.

Faith as a risk factor

Religious expression giving cause for concern in relation to mental health can include:

- excessive worship
- selective, repeated use of religious language, imagery or symbolism
- a person's belief that she is a particular (usually significant) religious figure (e.g. Joan of Arc), or that she has been entrusted with a mission to save the world
- a belief in demonic or spirit possession.

The idea that religion promotes unreasonable and sometimes health-damaging levels of guilt or shame is a popular one in the mental health context. Existing feelings of guilt might attract individuals to religions that preach doctrines of sin and forgiveness. More women than men experience strong guilt feelings and they are more likely to be 'intropunitive', which means tending to blame oneself. This could explain their greater religiosity.

There is a theory that most of us think in images, and we often bring childhood images of God unquestioningly into our adult lives, where they can be unhelpful. During times of distress, images of God can reappear in a powerful and disturbing way, often because they no longer rest well with a woman's emotional world. Although favourable God images can enhance self-esteem, improve life adjustment and promote positive health outcomes, the reverse is true for negative images. Specific male images of God, and the attribution of masculine characteristics to God, can be quite disturbing for women, particularly for those who have experienced sexual abuse or male oppression in their lives.

Negative images can mask an inability to know how to respond to everyday life situations in which a woman feels unsupported or lost. Painful feelings concerning perceived abandonment by a deity can lead to self-blame and a lessened sense of personal responsibility and agency. It is important for women to be creative in understanding and unpicking the images of God/Other they hold, and to pursue images that are positive in terms of their well-being as an alternative to images that are more negative.

Conclusions

Spiritual/religious beliefs and the use of religious imagery, especially during times of disturbance, can be viewed as 'vehicles' expressing other, deeper truths about the person. They are additional ways of understanding and discovering what might be going on in a woman's life, and perhaps the conflicts that could be causing or contributing to a problem.

Useful resources

National Spirituality and Mental Health Forum
www.mhspirituality.org.uk
The Forum aims to foster links between faith communities nationwide and the world of mental health.

Royal College of Psychiatrists' Spirituality and Psychiatry Special Interest Group
www.rcpsych.ac.uk/college/specialinterestgroups/spirituality.aspx
This special interest group was formed to explore the influence of the major religions. There is a vast publications archive on the website that is a valuable resource for anyone wishing to find out more about the interaction of spirituality/religion and mental health.

Spiritual Crisis Network
www.spiritualcrisisnetwork.org.uk
The Network promotes understanding and support for those going through profound personal transformation.

St Marylebone Healing and Counselling Centre
http://marylebone-hcc.org.uk
The Centre offers a number of approaches to healing, including professional counselling and psychotherapy, a mental health support group, spiritual direction and healing prayer. It also offers conferences about psychotherapy and spirituality, arts workshops, a consultation service for health professionals, and supervision groups.

References and further reading

Beit-Hallahmi B, Argyle M (1997) *The Psychology of Religious Behaviour, Belief and Experience*. Routledge.

Egan KJ, Cunningham LS (1996) *Christian Spirituality: Themes From the Tradition*. Paulist Press.

Fallot R, Heckman J (2005) Religious/spiritual coping among women trauma survivors with mental health and substance use disorders. *Journal of Behavioural Health Services and Research*, **32**, 215–226.

Helminiak D (1996) *The Human Core of Spirituality: Mind as Psyche and Spirit*. State University of New York Press.

Hood R, Spilka B, Hunsberger B, *et al* (1996) *The Psychology of Religion: An Empirical Approach*. Guilford Press.

Koenig H (ed.) (1998) *Handbook of Religion and Mental Health.* Academic Press.

Koenig H, Pargament K, Nielsen J (1998) Religious coping and health status in medically ill hospitalized older adults. *Journal of Nervous and Mental Disorders,* **186**, 513–521.

Lonsdale D (2000) *Spiritual Direction and Mental Health.* Bishop John Robinson.

Maton K (1989) The stress-buffering role of spiritual support: cross-sectional and prospective investigations. *Journal of the Scientific Study of Religion,* **28**, 310–323.

Paloutzian R (1996) *Invitation to the Psychology of Religion.* Allyn & Bacon.

Pargament KI, Park CL (1995) Merely a defense? The variety of religious means and ends. *Journal of Social Issues,* **51**, 13–32.

Pargament K, Ensing D, Falgout K, *et al* (1990) God help me: (I): religious coping efforts as predictors of the outcomes to significant negative life events. *American Journal of Community Psychology,* **18**, 793–824.

Reid-Arndt S, Smith M, Yoon DP, *et al* (2011) Gender differences in spiritual experiences, religious practices, and congregational support for individuals with significant health conditions. *Journal of Religion, Disability and Health,* **15**, 175–196.

Rizzuto A (1981) *The Birth of the Living God: A Psychoanalytic Study.* University of Chicago Press.

Schumaker J (ed.) (1992) *Religion and Mental Health.* Oxford University Press.

Sims A, Cook C (2009) Spirituality in psychiatry. In *Spirituality and Psychiatry* (eds C Cook, A Powell & A Sims). RCPsych Publications.

Trzebiatowska M, Bruce S (2012) *Why are Women More Religious than Men?* Oxford Scholarship Online.

Vahia I, Depp C, Palmer B, *et al* (2011) Correlates of spirituality in older women. *Aging and Mental Health,* **15**, 97–102.

Linking physical and mental health in women

Irene Cormac

Women have a key role in managing their own and their family's health. This chapter outlines some of the factors that affect women's health and recommends ways to improve it.

Women's health

In the UK, life expectancy has risen over the past 100 years. In part, this is due to better disease prevention and improved detection and treatment of diseases. In 2016, the average life expectancy of a 65-year-old woman rose to 86 years (Public Health England, 2016). Life expectancy tends to be greater in more affluent areas than in poorer areas. Causes of death in the UK vary with age group. In women aged 20–34 years the leading cause of death is suicide (12% of deaths); in ages 35–49 years it is breast cancer (14% of deaths) and in women over 80 years it is dementia (17% of deaths) (ONS, 2015).

Compared with men, women tend to be shorter, have less muscle mass and blood, and have smaller lung, liver and kidney capacities. This means that women are more sensitive to the harmful effects of smoking and alcohol, and side-effects of medicine. Reproductive health plays a part, too. Young women are more at risk of sexually transmitted diseases. On the positive side, rates of teenage pregnancy have recently fallen to their lowest recorded levels (ONS, 2017).

Linking physical and mental health

Physical conditions can cause mental health problems

It is essential to discover whether a physical condition is causing a mental problem or illness, because the treatment will be different. For example, is some medicine taken to treat severe acne causing a young person's depression? Is an overactive thyroid gland causing anxiety and weight loss? Is depression and psychosis due to an underactive thyroid gland? Is delirium causing a confused state or does the person have dementia, or both conditions? Simple blood tests can be used to screen for many of the physical causes of mental health conditions.

Mental health conditions can worsen physical health

In the UK, 30% of those with long-term physical conditions also have mental health conditions (4.6 million people) (Naylor *et al*, 2012). For instance, depression can complicate illnesses such as diabetes mellitus. Depression increases the risk three-fold that a patient will not take their medical treatment (Di Matteo *et al*, 2000) which would compromise their recovery.

Severe mental illness can shorten life

Research has shown that women with all forms of mental disorder lose between 9.8 and 17.5 life-years, compared with their expected length of life; schizoaffective disorders lead to the most loss of life-years (Chang *et al*, 2011). Eating disorders such as anorexia nervosa can compromise physical health and increase the risk of dying prematurely fivefold; addictions also cause poor physical and mental health, leading to a fourfold increase in risk of premature death (Harris & Barraclough, 1998). Side-effects of some medicines used to treat mental illness can also compromise physical health.

Factors that determine health

Different health risk factors affect the risk of dying prematurely to a different extent (Box 13.1).

Behavioural patterns that affect health include inactivity, tobacco smoking, poor diet and obesity, drinking alcohol above recommended limits and taking recreational drugs. Risky sexual behaviour increases the risk of contracting sexually transmitted diseases and of unwanted pregnancy.

Genetic susceptibility to illness is set in a person's genetic make-up at conception. Genetic mapping has been used to

---

Box 13.1   Health risks and dying prematurely

- Behavioural patterns (40%)
- Genetic risk factors (30%)
- Social circumstances (15%)
- Healthcare (10%)
- Environmental exposure (5%)

The figures are for women and men. Source: Schroeder (2007).

---

identify sites on the human genome that cause or affect various physical and mental conditions. Two genetic mutations (abnormal genes) occur in about 1 in 10 women with breast cancer – breast cancer genes 1 and 2 (*BRCA1* and *BRCA2*). There is often a history of breast cancer in close female relatives in those carrying these genes. Women who know they are (or could be) carrying genes that might increase the risk to their offspring of inheriting a disease or disability can seek genetic screening and counselling.

Social risk factors for health are often outside an individual's control. Adverse social circumstances include living in poverty, living in poor housing, being unemployed, having a poor education and lacking social protection. Government and social policies can address social inequalities, education and provision of social care, and organisations such as Citizens Advice, charities and the police can provide help and advice to those experiencing domestic violence and abuse.

In the UK, healthcare is provided by the National Health Service (NHS), plus private and charitable healthcare providers. With increasing pressures on healthcare, one of the challenges is to prevent disease and disability in the general population, so that people not only live longer but also enjoy healthier lives. Women need to continue to have access to good obstetric and family planning services. People with mental health problems should have access to the same standard of physical healthcare as people without these conditions.

Environmental exposures to health risks include air pollution, contaminated water and risks from living in neighbourhoods with high levels of violence. Overcrowding contributes to the spread of infectious diseases such as influenza and tuberculosis.

Infectious diseases include HIV, sexually transmitted diseases and viruses (e.g. the human papillomavirus (HPV) that causes cancer of the cervix and the tongue). Women need to be aware of the signs of developing cancer – 'red flag' symptoms – and if any are noticed, medical advice should be sought (Table 13.1).

Table 13.1   Cancer 'red flags': symptoms to look out for

Symptoms	Cancer
• Cough for more than 3 weeks • Blood in coughed-up sputum	Lung
• Changes in bowel habits • Blood in stools	Bowel
• Lump in the breast • Change in breast shape • Discharge from the nipple	Breast
• Persistently bloated stomach • Abdominal or pelvic pain	Ovary
• Fits • Headaches • Nausea • Weakness • Vision problems	Brain

Tips on how to improve and maintain health

- Adults aged 19–64 should exercise for at least 150 min (moderate activity) per week, and do strength exercises two or more days a week (advice from NHS Choices).
- Eat a Mediterranean diet and manage weight to reduce the risk of developing diabetes and heart disease. There is evidence that the risk of dementia can be reduced by diet, and by physical and mental exercises (see the FINGER study by Ngandu *et al* (2015)).
- Immunisation protects against infections such as influenza and meningitis, and the HPV vaccine protects against cervical cancer.
- Avoid risky sex by using contraception and barriers to infection.

- Reduce social health risks by avoiding loneliness if possible and by applying for benefits when experiencing financial hardship.
- Check for bodily changes, for example, self-check breasts.
- Take part in health screening (e.g. mammograms, cervical screen, bowel cancer screening) and, when relevant, screening for complications of chronic diseases, for instance diabetes mellitus.
- Register with a general practitioner and dentist. Seek help for mental and physical health issues, domestic violence and abuse.
- Be aware of the side-effects of medicines.

References and further reading

Chang C-K, Hayes RD, Perera G, *et al* (2011) Life expectancy at birth for people with serious mental illness and other major disorders from a secondary mental health care case register in London. *PLoS ONE*, **6**, e19590.

DiMatteo MR, Lepper HS, Crogham TW (2000) Depression is a risk factor for non-compliance with medical treatment. *Archives of Internal Medicine*, **160**, 2101–2107.

Harris EC, Barraclough B (1998) Excess mortality of mental disorder. *British Journal of Psychiatry*, **173**, 11–53.

Naylor C, Parsonage M, McDaid D, *et al* (2012) *Long-Term Conditions and Mental Health: The Cost of Co-Morbidities*. The King's Fund/Centre For Mental Health.

Ngandu T, Lehtisalo J, Solomon A, *et al* (2015) A 2-year multidomain intervention of diet, exercise, cognitive training, and vascular risk monitoring versus control to prevent cognitive decline in at-risk elderly people (FINGER): a randomised controlled trial. *Lancet*, **385**, 2255–2263.

NHS Choices (2017) Physical activity guidelines for adults. Available at http://www.nhs.uk/Livewell/fitness/Pages/physical-activity-guidelines-for-adults.aspx (accessed 21 May 2017).

Office for National Statistics (2015) What are the top causes of death by age and gender? ONS. Available at http://visual.ons.gov.uk/what-are-the-top-causes-of-death-by-age-and-gender/ (accessed 21 May 2017).

Office for National Statistics (2017) *Statistical Bulletin: Conceptions in England and Wales: 2015*. ONS.

Public Health England (2016) *Life Expectancy: Recent Trends in Older Ages PHE* (Publications Gateway Number: 2015661). PHE.

Schroeder SA (2007) We can do better – improving the health of the American people. *New England Journal of Medicine*, **357**, 1221–1228.

Obesity

John Morgan

In ancient times, the human brain adapted to manage hunger. Women in particular became exquisitely attuned to cycles of feast and famine, with fertility switched on by feast and switched off by famine. Food became a reward, an antidepressant and a comfort. Female beauty and female health became entwined in cultural ideals.

Now, many of us live in an urban jungle. We move less and eat more. Even in the developing world, obesity is outstripping underweight. Hunger drives our behaviour more strongly than satiety, and a powerful food industry encourages greater consumption of saturated fats and dairy products than ever before. No wonder we face an obesity epidemic.

But weight is more complex than that. Only a quarter of schoolgirls are actually overweight, but two-thirds believe they are. Body image disparagement is widespread and girls face counterproductive social pressures to lose weight and reshape their bodies. The female beauty ideal is divorced from female health, leaving many women and girls at war with their bodies. So there is more to tackling obesity than simply moving more and eating less.

For many overweight women, psychological factors are as relevant as they are for women with anorexia or bulimia nervosa. Research has shown that 'pleasure centres' in the brain light up with the mere thought of food, and food can be as addictive as alcohol and cigarettes. But whereas women with alcohol problems can avoid going to pubs and bars, and drug addicts can hide their illness from prying eyes, for the obese, there is no avoiding food. The stigma is always visible. Overweight women are demonised and society equates female restraint with moral virtue.

Countering obesity

So what is to be done? There is no one-size-fits-all solution. Society has tackled smoking and alcohol misuse through public health policies on advertising and taxation. But the food industry is a powerful lobby group.

We need to promote positive, diverse body image and healthy living in schools, turning away from an excessive focus on weight and guiding children to strong self-esteem through healthy behaviours. Prevention is better than cure, and our children are harmed by scare stories about obesity that trigger unsustainable, counterproductive diets.

Behavioural change works for many. Small, sustainable lifestyle changes are better than faddish diets. We achieve such change through motivation and self-knowledge. Measuring behaviour and diet allows for small shifts in behaviour, such as eating more fresh fruit and vegetables, or taking modest amounts of regular exercise. Self-monitoring, including monitoring emotions, can be done offline and online, in the pages of a book or electronically.

Support groups provide encouragement and motivation to keep going through inevitable success and failure. Commercial support groups are successful and popular because they work for the many. More personalised, tailor-made treatment programmes are even more effective, including nutritional and emotional analysis, motivational enhancement therapy and psychological formulation. Relatively modest weight loss can lead to huge health benefits. For example, a 5% weight loss improves metabolic morbidity.

Surgery

Some women need medical or surgical treatments. Women should only use medication as part of a holistic approach to weight loss. The benefits are clear, but also modest.

In morbid obesity, surgery (known as bariatric surgery) produces sustained benefits. Over the past decade, research has examined treatment outcomes in morbid obesity. For example, the Yorkshire Nutrition and Obesity Team (Y-NOT) has shown that psychological factors are strong predictors of the success of physical treatments of morbid obesity. Emotion-driven eating will not necessarily stop as a result of physical constraints, and can get worse.

Overweight women can benefit from bariatric surgery when obesity occurs alongside other health conditions, such as polycystic ovary syndrome, infertility, diabetes, high blood pressure and abnormal breathing and waking at night because of obesity (known as sleep apnoea; see Chapter 15). However, there must be evidence of previous weight-loss attempts, acceptance of the risks of surgery and an ability to comply with post-operative behavioural change.

Psychological therapy

Psychological therapy is rarely sufficient to achieve sustained weight loss, but it lays the foundations for other treatments. For people who are obese with binge-eating disorder, bulimia nervosa, undertreated depression or unresolved trauma, psychological therapies are crucial before lifestyle changes, medications or surgery can have an effect. Eating disorder specialists provide psychological understanding of what drives the condition and therapy that permits longer-term solutions.

Conclusions

Obesity treatment aims for weight maintenance in the first instance. It requires access to expertise, including body image therapies, individualised lifestyle interventions and medication, and in women who are eligible the final treatment option is bariatric surgery.

There have been many false dawns in the history of obesity treatment. For most women who are overweight, individualised therapies focused on behavioural change result in small victories that transform the woman's quality of life, even when weight loss is less than expected. However, for a significant minority, obesity is as psychologically complex as anorexia nervosa. Every day, cognitive neuroscience is helping us to form a deeper understanding of how to reprogramme our love–hate relationship with food.

Women and sleep

Neil Stanley

Sleep is a biological necessity and good sleep is essential for good physical, mental and emotional health. Women's sleep is affected in different ways compared with men's because of biological and psychosocial influences, and women's sleep changes at different stages of their lives. Sleep disorders in women are often overlooked by doctors: for example, sleep-disordered breathing is commonly associated with middle-aged men, but around 10% of women also suffer from it.

Insomnia and mental health problems often go together. Poor sleep has been linked with an increased risk of depression and anxiety and, in turn, insomnia is common in both anxiety and depression (Neckelmann *et al*, 2007).

Stages of sleep

Sleep is divided into two distinct states: rapid eye movement (REM) sleep and non-REM sleep. Non-REM sleep is further divided into three stages. During the night you pass through the four sleep stages (1, 2, 3 and REM sleep) in what are known as sleep cycles. Each cycle lasts an average of 90–110 min. The first sleep cycles of the night have long periods of deep sleep and relatively short periods of REM sleep. Later in the night, however, the periods of REM sleep lengthen and deep sleep is mostly absent.

Stage 1 sleep

Stage 1 sleep (3–7% of sleep) is the lightest stage of sleep and is the transition between wake and sleep. The eyes move slowly back and forth and muscle activity reduces.

Stage 2 sleep

In Stage 2 sleep (45–50% of sleep), the slow, rolling eye movements seen in Stage 1 sleep stop. Brain waves become slower, with only occasional bursts of rapid brain waves.

Stage 3 sleep

In Stage 3 sleep (25% of sleep), sleep becomes deeper and extremely slow brain waves (called delta waves) appear. This is the deepest, most restorative stage of sleep and is most closely linked with the part sleep plays in making us feel well-rested and energetic during the day. Deep sleep is also important for memory and learning.

REM sleep

In REM sleep (20–25% of sleep), the eyes jerk rapidly back and forth under closed eyelids (hence its name). It is during REM sleep that most story-like dreams occur. Everyone dreams every night, and we have three to five periods of REM sleep each night. However, we can only remember a dream if we are woken during it or within a couple of minutes after it has finished. REM sleep is involved in processing emotional memories and ensuring our psychological health.

Sleep disturbances in young women

In general, women sleep best in their 20s, but sleep disturbances often occur with the menstrual cycle, pregnancy and motherhood. It has become increasingly common for young women to live a fast-paced lifestyle, which means that they often neglect their need for sleep.

Menstrual cycle

The hormones oestrogen and progesterone, which have a role in regulating the menstrual cycle, can also influence sleep and circadian rhythms. Many women report 2–3 days of disrupted sleep during each cycle.

Some women experience more awakenings and other sleep disturbances during their premenstrual period, while other women report excessive sleepiness, fatigue and longer sleeping hours. Premenstrual symptoms such as food cravings and emotional changes can also directly affect women's sleep. Significant sleep disruption has been reported in association with premenstrual syndrome or premenstrual dysphoric disorder (a severe form of premenstrual syndrome affecting 3–8% of women).

For some women, sleep problems are a by-product of other menstrual symptoms (e.g. abdominal cramping, bloating, headaches and breast tenderness) or dysmenorrhoea (painful menstruation). Oral contraceptives affect body temperature regulation and this can also affect sleep. Women on oral contraceptives have more Stage 2 sleep and less of the restful, restorative, deep sleep.

Pregnancy

Pregnancy substantially disrupts sleep, with up to 75% of women having problems with insomnia at this time. Most women report daytime fatigue and the need for longer night-time sleep. Altered sleep during early pregnancy may relate to nausea and vomiting during the first trimester. Stress linked to first-time or unplanned pregnancies or the absence of good psychosocial support can also cause insomnia.

During later pregnancy, the time spent asleep decreases and sleep quality gets worse. During the second and third trimesters, waking at night, fatigue, leg cramps, difficulty sleeping in certain positions and shortness of breath become more common.

Pregnant women who experience sleep disturbances should think about symptoms of depression, as disrupted sleep might indicate an underlying change in mood. Pregnant women, especially during the final trimester, are more likely to have sleep apnoea (see 'Obstructive sleep apnoea' below) and restless legs syndrome (RLS). Snoring also increases during pregnancy (14–45% of pregnant women *v.* 4% of non-pregnant women).

Motherhood

Sleep is often disturbed in motherhood. In the early years, this disturbance is caused by the different sleep and feeding patterns of the child. In the later years, the combinaton of the responsibilities of motherhood with other roles can lead to stress and neglect of sleep hygiene, as women prioritise daytime activities over night-time sleep.

Sleep disturbances in older women

Menopause

During menopause, 25–50% of women experience sleep disturbances. In particular, hot flushes and night sweats cause repeated waking owing to the sensation of heat and sweating, as well as an increased heart rate and anxiety. Because the sleep disturbance is related to room temperature, it is important to have a cool temperature in the bedroom with light, cotton bed linen, and to avoid anything that also raises body temperature before bed. Hormone replacement therapy can improve sleep by relieving severe hot flushes.

Post-menopause

In the years following the menopause, sleep naturally becomes lighter and more easily disturbed, making it more difficult to maintain uninterrupted sleep and to feel refreshed during the day. Other physical factors also become more common, including arthritis, chronic lung disease, certain medications, heartburn, anxiety and frequent urination – these can also disturb sleep.

Insomnia

Insomnia is the most common sleep problem, and is almost twice as common in women as in men. Sometimes, women begin to have sleepless nights associated with menstruation, pregnancy or menopause and then find it difficult to break poor sleep habits. If insomnia persists and lifestyle, behavioural or diet changes do not help, a doctor may prescribe a sleep-promoting medication. In some instances, there may be an underlying and treatable cause, such as depression (women are twice as likely to report depression as men), stress, anxiety, reflux, bladder problems or pain. If these conditions are appropriately treated, there should be an improvement in sleep.

Chronic insomnia is also a risk factor for developing anxiety and depression (Neckelmann *et al*, 2007).

Obstructive sleep apnoea

Obstructive sleep apnoea is a serious sleep disorder characterised by snoring, interrupted breathing during sleep and excessive daytime sleepiness. It is more common in pregnant women, particularly during the final trimester, and has been associated with conditions such as pre-eclampsia/high blood pressure, gestational diabetes and poor growth of the fetus. (Even snoring has been linked with adverse pregnancy outcomes.)

Obstructive sleep apnoea is generally less common in women than men, but becomes more common in women over the age of 50. Because being overweight is a risk factor for sleep apnoea, and women tend to increase their abdominal fat during the menopause, menopausal women become more likely to develop this sleep disorder. Menopausal women also have a diminishing level of progesterone, which is a respiratory stimulant. The main treatments for obstructive sleep apnoea are weight loss and a reduction in alcohol and any sedative medications that are being taken.

Restless legs syndrome

RLS is a neurological movement disorder involving unpleasant feelings, usually in the legs. Because these unpleasant feelings occur at rest and are relieved by movement, RLS sufferers often have difficulty sleeping.

Up to 10% of adults have this condition and it is twice as common in women as in men. Over 75% of those with RLS also have periodic limb movement disorder, which involves involuntary leg twitching or jerking movements during sleep that can occur every 20–30 s.

Deficiencies in dietary requirements, especially iron, are likely to play a part in RLS. It is extremely common in pregnancy, being reported by up to 50% of pregnant women, particularly during the third trimester, which may be linked to anaemia (lack of iron in the blood) at this time. Iron and/or vitamin B12 supplements, cold/warm compresses, massage and avoiding caffeine, nicotine and alcohol can improve RLS.

Shift work

Many women do shift work. Shift workers generally report more sleep-related accidents and illnesses. Women who work night shifts get less sleep and their sleep is more disturbed. Difficulty falling asleep and obtaining quality sleep during the day hours is a common problem in these women.

Night and rotating shifts can put a strain on family life, as less time is available to meet home responsibilities and enjoy recreational and social activities. Female shift workers are also more likely to experience irregular menstrual cycles, difficulty getting pregnant, higher rates of miscarriage, premature births and low-birth-weight babies. Changes in exposure to light and lost sleep caused by shift work can have significant biological or hormonal effects. There is conflicting evidence concerning the association between shift work and an increased risk of breast cancer.

Tips for getting better sleep

- It is important to go to bed with a quiet mind and relaxed body.
- Your bedroom should be dark, quiet and cool.
- The bedroom should be strongly associated with sleep, so if you are not going to sleep you should not be in your bedroom. This means no TV, no computer and no work in the bedroom.
- Go to bed only when you're sleepy. This means listening to your body rather than going to bed because you've finished watching TV, or because your partner wants to go to bed, etc.
- If you don't fall asleep within about 30 min at the start of the night, get up and only go back to bed again when you are sleepy (if you wake up in the middle of the night and do not fall asleep within around 20 min, do the same).
- Don't clock-watch. Close your eyes to encourage yourself to sleep.
- Try to have a regular bedtime and wake-up time.
- Do not worry about your sleep and do not 'try' to go to sleep. The harder you 'try' to sleep the less likely you are to fall asleep.

- Try to spend at least 30 min winding down before bed. Put the worries and cares of the day aside and do something nice and relaxing.
- Remember, you cannot find sleep, sleep must find you.

Useful resources

American Academy of Sleep Medicine
www.sleepeducation.com

British Snoring and Sleep Apnoea Association
www.britishsnoring.co.uk

References and further reading

Attarian HP, Viola-Saltzman M (eds) (2013) *Sleep Disorders in Women: A Guide to Practical Management* (2nd edn). Humana Press.

Kryger M (2004) *A Woman's Guide to Sleep Disorders*. McGraw–Hill Professional.

Moline ML, Broch L, Zak R, *et al* (2003) Sleep in women across the life cycle from adulthood through menopause. *Sleep Medicine Reviews*, **7**, 155–177.

Neckelmann D, Mykletun A, Dahl AA (2007) Chronic insomnia as a risk factor for developing anxiety and depression. *Sleep*, **30**, 873–880.

Women and pain

George Ikkos and Susan Lingwood

Imani's story

Imani is a 33-year-old medical secretary. She is a quiet, introverted person with no family and few friends, working in a department with a lot of stress. One day she had a minor injury to her knee. Surprisingly, she developed severe pain in her whole leg, with swelling and temperature and colour changes. Her general practitioner (GP) and doctors at the accident and emergency service (A&E) thought she was making up her symptoms, but she became increasingly disabled until, finally, she was unable to walk. A specialist in pain medicine assessed her, and diagnosed her with chronic regional pain syndrome. The doctor gave her medication to control the pain and she started a rehabilitation programme that made a big difference to how she was feeling. This allowed Imani to return to work, though some pain and colour changes returned from time to time.

Pain, especially acute pain, is often useful. It warns us that a part of our body is injured or at risk of being damaged. Without the experience of pain, we would not know to take our hand from the fire or attend to a broken leg. However, pain can also signal a false alarm. For example, headache, the most common pain, is not usually associated with any actual damage to the head or brain. Usually it is caused by spasms in the muscles around the head and neck. It is, however, important to attend to pain as a warning sign. Pain can be a physical or a psychological warning sign, and is most often a combination of both. Pain is well recognised to be more common in women, partly because of the fact that only women experience menstrual pain and pain during labour.

It is important to understand both the physical and the psychological aspects of pain. A lack of awareness of the psychological side leads patients and doctors to rely excessively on medication and other physical treatments such as injections or surgery. It is now well established that the overprescription of medication for pain can do more harm than good. Of course, the judicious prescription of medication and, in selected cases, injections or even surgery, can be helpful.

The double nature of pain

Physical aspects of pain

Sarah's story

Sarah is a 32-year-old teacher who needed to be induced early in her first pregnancy. She had heard horror stories from friends about childbirth and was expecting medical intervention to be necessary. By talking through her fears about labour realistically with close friends and learning about relaxation and breathing techniques, she entered the hospital in a relatively calm state. Her labour progressed quickly, and although she requested epidural analgesia, this was not possible in time. She eventually gave birth naturally to a healthy baby the following day. On reflection, she felt that the pain was 'awful', 'the worst ever', but she had managed it, knowing that this was 'normal' and her new baby was on his way.

Pain is normally generated by chemical substances in parts of the body, whether external (e.g. the fingers) or internal (e.g. the gut), where there is a harmful change or the risk of a harmful change. In Sarah's case, the contractions of the womb and passage of the fetus through the birth canal caused extreme pain, which is nonetheless manageable by millions of women worldwide, and in which the use of medication and injections has been very helpful.

The chemical messages created by the painful stimulus (e.g. stretching of tissues, damage to skin) are transmitted along our nervous system, all the way to the brain, where we also interpret the pain with our emotions and thoughts. In Sarah's example, the pain felt manageable because the cause (childbirth) was well understood and, although fearful, she felt well supported by the obstetric team.

Surprisingly, perhaps, when pain is more long-lasting (chronic), it can feel more painful. Research has shown that chronic pain makes the central nervous system even more sensitive to pain (Woolf, 2011). There are two ways this happens.

- In the 'wind-up' phenomenon, the nerve fibres specialising in pain become more sensitive because of chemical changes. This can cause hyperalgesia, in which the pain sensation is much stronger than would normally be associated with that particular stimulus. The effect is like holding a magnifying lens to the pain.
- In 'central sensitisation', nerve fibres that are normally not responsive to pain become sensitive. For example, nerve fibres that normally respond to light touch start causing us to feel pain. This is known as 'allodynia'.

Both these experiences happen primarily through physical, not psychological, processes. Although hyperalgesia and allodynia are distressing, they are not a sign that nerves, muscles, joints or other parts of the body are becoming more damaged.

Psychological aspects of pain

Naz's story

Naz is a 56-year-old hairdresser with a successful business. She works long hours through a busy schedule, despite suffering vague aches and pains from time to time; she is drinking a little too much to cope with the pressures of work and family, and is not sleeping well. One day she woke up with severe back pain. She could not understand why, because she had not had an accident, so far as she could remember. When Naz called her GP, she was asked to complete a simple questionnaire and then she had a sensitive conversation with her doctor. It turned out that Naz had become increasingly depressed over the past few months since she had discovered that her husband was having an affair, and she had not been able to tell anyone. X-rays and scans did not show any abnormality in her back and she improved with counselling and antidepressant medication. Within a couple of months she had hardly any pain.

Psychological factors can have a big influence on pain. They can help relieve pain, but they can also cause it, make it worse, keep it going or bring it back after it has stopped. As in Naz's case, stress from family or work can cause back pain (or headache or neck pain), as well as other physical symptoms. Focusing on and worrying excessively about pain (why is this happening? what is wrong with me?) can exacerbate it, whether it is a stress-induced headache or pain caused by a physical problem such as arthritis. Conversely, distraction and engagement in rewarding activities, including appropriate exercise, may limit the intensity, duration and effects of pain.

It might be helpful to think of two pain pathways going from the spinal cord to the brain. One goes to the sensory cortex, which tells us where the pain is and how strong it is. The other pathway goes to the limbic system. This is a more primitive part of our brain. It is the emotional engine of the nervous system and tells us how upsetting and distressing the pain is. Worry, fear, anxiety, depression, enjoyment and reward influence the limbic system, which is why psychological factors can have a big effect on our experience of pain.

Our relationships, home life, culture and the society we live in also have a part to play in how we respond to and manage pain. The way our caregivers have responded to us in childhood, soothing us when injured, or reassuring us when hurt, influences how we understand pain and how we respond to it as adults. For example, if we witnessed a relative suffering with a chronic disabling illness, it is not surprising that when faced with similar pain we may become worried about it. This can make the pain worse, and influences how we go about seeking help and managing our health.

The way we change our behaviour, once pain starts, influences its strength and duration. For example, women who give up exercise because of back or other pain will experience deconditioning of their body, particularly of their muscles. This in itself causes pain, even when not exercising. Being out of condition also makes people experience more pain when they start exercising again. It is important not to feel alarmed when this happens and to consider doing a little bit at a time, rather than overdoing it on a 'good' day. The concept of pacing is very important here. When in doubt, ask a doctor or other clinical specialist.

Managing pain

There are many different types of pain and the best way to manage them will vary. Gut (stomach) pain that is caused by irritable bowel syndrome (IBS) might require simple dietary advice or lifestyle changes, whereas similar pain from ulcerative colitis will require strong medication and sometimes even surgery. A new, acute (short-term) pain will need different management from a familiar, chronic pain. The good news is that simple measures help the majority of pain and certain approaches will help regardless of the cause of chronic pain.

Many clinics run pain management programmes using the principles of cognitive–behavioural therapy (CBT). CBT is a psychological therapy that focuses on changing the way we think, feel and behave to improve how we manage our symptoms. CBT is now widely available in the UK and can be accessed as self-help (using a book or online resource, such as www.llttf.com), as one-to-one talking therapy with a health professional, or through group work (self-refer to your local Improving Access to Psychological Therapies (IAPT) service) (Morley *et al*, 1999). Another effective approach is mindfulness-based stress reduction. The idea is to learn to observe and attend to the sensations experienced in the body, and gain some distance from them. Many patients have benefited from this approach, which can also help reduce depression and anxiety (Kabat-Zinn, 1982; Grossman *et al*, 2004).

Apart from these two examples, there are many other self-help and psychological approaches to pain (see 'Useful resources' at the end of this chapter). As well as psychological approaches, sometimes taking antidepressant medication can be helpful, even if you are not feeling depressed. This is best to discuss with a GP or pain specialist.

GPs and anaesthetists are the main medical professionals who deal with pain. For more complex or chronic pain (if simple measures have not helped enough), anaesthetists who specialise in pain, often in multidisciplinary teams with physiotherapists and occupational therapists, can be helpful. These teams can also include psychologists and sometimes psychiatrists, and offer pain management programmes. Choosing a specialist is best done with advice from a GP and taking into account other symptoms and any history of pain.

Tips for a woman experiencing pain

- The best outcomes depend on a trusting relationship between patient and doctor and a collaborative approach.

- Often, even the best doctors may not be able to locate a specific physical cause for pain or other symptoms. In this case, it is crucial that you feel the doctor has listened to you and that you can accept the doctor's reassurance.
- Do not worry unnecessarily and obsessively about your health as this may even prolong or exacerbate the pain.
- When a doctor says they can find no physical cause for the pain, it does not mean they do not believe in it or that there is no need for help to manage it.
- Sometimes when there does not seem to be a physical cause for the pain, it may be primarily due to a psychological or psychiatric problem. You may benefit greatly from a psychiatrist's or psychologist's opinion.
- Psychiatrists who specialise in pain may have other medications or treatments to recommend and these can make a huge difference, even for women whose problems have seemed intractable.

Useful resources

The British Pain Society
www.britishpainsociety.org

Living Life to the Full
www.llttf.com

Neurosymptoms.org
www.neurosymptoms.org

References and further reading

Grossman P, Niemann L, Schmidt S, *et al* (2004) Mindfulness-based stress reduction and health benefits: a meta-analysis. *Journal of Psychosomatic Research*, **57**, 35–43.

Kabat-Zinn J (1982) An outpatient program in behavioral medicine for chronic pain patients based on the practice of mindfulness meditation: theoretical considerations and preliminary results. *General Hospital Psychiatry*, **4**, 33–47.

Morley S, Eccleston C, Williams A (1999) Systematic review and meta-analysis of randomised controlled trials of cognitive behaviour therapy and behaviour therapy for chronic pain in adults, excluding headache. *Pain*, **80**, 1–13.

Woolf CJ (2011) Central sensitization: implications for the diagnosis and treatment of pain. *Pain*, **152** (Suppl 3), S2–S15.

Bereavement, loss and grief

Lynne M. Drummond

Gladys's story

Gladys is an 82-year-old woman who had been married to Bert for over 60 years when he died suddenly of a heart attack. Following the death, her two sons arrived and stayed nearby, helping her with the funeral arrangements and sorting through his effects. Gladys lived in Leeds, her eldest son lived in London and her younger son lived in Glasgow. Immediately following the death, they were amazed at how well she seemed to be coping, noting that she was still smiling and very pleased to see them. Indeed, they were so encouraged with her apparent coping ability that they all returned to their homes after 3 weeks with no concerns about her. As before, they telephoned her once a week.

Three months after Bert's death, George received a telephone call from one of his mother's friends. She had become increasingly concerned that she had not seen Gladys since the funeral. Previously, Gladys had been a sociable lady who took part in various church activities, but she had not attended any social events or been seen in church since the funeral. Most of her friends had assumed she was staying with one of her sons. George was shocked to hear this and decided to travel to visit his mother the following week.

When he arrived, he could immediately see how overgrown the garden had become. His parents had always been keen gardeners, but now there was a mass of weeds and the grass was uncut. His mother was slow to answer the door and when she did, George was appalled to see how thin and unkempt she appeared, and how dirty and untidy the house was. Gladys had always been house proud and taken pride in her appearance. She was surprised to see George but welcomed him indoors and started general 'small talk' as she would do in her weekly telephone calls. It was clear that there was little food in the house and that Gladys had been mostly existing on bread and butter. George told his mother he would spend some time with her looking after some of the practical issues:

going shopping, helping clean the house, going through unopened mail, cutting the lawn and arranging for help with the garden. As they worked on these tasks, Gladys started to talk about how much she missed Bert and how empty her life felt without him. She felt unable to go out with friends as she did not wish them to see her the way she was.

Once she started talking, George could see she looked better. However, he was concerned that if he left her, she would revert to her depressed state. Gladys refused to visit her general practitioner (GP) as she felt she 'didn't want to bother the doctor with something like this'. George wanted to help his mother, but needed to return to his own family. He saw an advertisement for Cruse Bereavement Care and called the number. They told him of a support group for widows of a similar age to his mother. Gladys initially refused to visit the Cruse support group but, with George's encouragement, she eventually agreed. Initially, she claimed it was unhelpful, but she agreed to return the following week.

With the support of Cruse, Gladys began to improve. She remained intermittently tearful and low, but was able to start to cope with her life and to start to think about what she was going to do with her life without Bert.

We all have to deal with loss and bereavement during our lives. As humans are a social species who rely on each other and form close family and social bonds, these losses are typically traumatic and painful. Women tend to experience these losses more often than men, as they live longer: there are more widows than widowers. It is also true that women are more likely to be the main carers for elderly parents or for disabled children, and might experience the void of a loss even more acutely as they might also have to readjust their role and occupation.

Grief typically follows the death of a family member or friend. However, a similar reaction and the psychological symptoms of loss can also follow other losses. These include obvious situations such as the death of a family pet or a miscarriage, but also the grief felt by children following the divorce of their parents, the loss of a lover or the loss of status following redundancy or retirement.

Stages of grief

An individual typically experiences a number of stages of grief as they start to comprehend and come to terms with their loss. Although I have described these as stages, not everyone will experience all of them, and they will not necessarily occur in the order given. Although I have stated the average length of time these stages last, this can also vary greatly between women and can depend on the emotional magnitude of the loss experienced. The stages are:

- disbelief and numbness
- yearning and trying to make sense of the loss
- depression and isolation
- acceptance and moving on.

Disbelief and numbness

Immediately following a loss, most women feel numb and as if the events that are occurring are unreal. To a casual observer, it might appear that the bereaved individual is acting in an uncaring or callous way, but in reality she is in a state of shock and denial. This state can last for a few hours or even days and can occur after expected as well as sudden, unexpected deaths.

Yearning and trying to make sense of the loss

When the numbness wears off, there can be waves of extreme yearning for the loved one. During this time there might be sudden outbursts of crying, symptoms of anxiety and panic, an inability to sleep, reduced appetite and loss of concentration. During this time, many women feel guilty about their relationship with their loved one, wishing they had spent more time with them or had had a better relationship with them (this reaction is common even in people who had a very good relationship with the deceased). Sometimes women feel extreme anger towards people whom they perceive, rightly or wrongly, to be responsible for the death. This anger can take the form of blaming the healthcare professionals involved in the care of the deceased, anger at other family members who they feel have not acted appropriately, or even anger at the person who has died. These thoughts and feelings often last for days or weeks. During this time, the bereaved woman might think she can see or hear her loved one. Some women describe how they feel the 'presence' of their loved ones.

Depression and isolation

Once the woman has fully accepted her loss, she might experience symptoms similar to depression. During this time she might feel sad and tearful, experience a lack of enjoyment in situations she had previously enjoyed, or feel a sense of futility. She might have reduced appetite, or comfort eat to try and overcome the emptiness and loss. Some women might isolate themselves and remove themselves from usual social situations. Others fail to engage fully with their work and other leisure activities. This stage can last for up to a year in some individuals.

Acceptance and moving on

Once the bereaved woman has accepted her loss, she can start to move on with her life. The scars of loss will inevitably still be there, but she can start to look forward to the future even without her loved one. Certain times like the anniversary of the death or the deceased person's birthday can cause a temporary re-emergence of feelings of loss.

Individual reactions to loss

Grief is a highly individualised experience and, although the stages listed are frequently experienced by many people, not all will be experienced by all.

Although there is considerable variability in grief symptoms, some types of death are more likely to result in complicated grief and prolonged mourning than others. In general, the death of a child or young person is more difficult than the death of an older person. Most of us expect to bury our parents, for example, but it is every mother's nightmare to outlive her child. Traumatic, violent or sudden deaths, and deaths by suicide, are often more difficult than deaths following ill health.

Although most women will overcome grief after a period of time without professional intervention, some can experience more lasting problems and need experienced help. Indications that professional help is needed include extreme, life-threatening symptoms, suicidal ideas, deep depression or symptoms that extend over more than a year without any evidence of resolution. This is known as complicated grief.

Treatment for complicated grief

There are two main approaches to the treatment of complicated grief:

- drug therapy
- psychological treatments.

In general, the drugs used to treat complicated grief work best on the symptoms of depression and low mood, rather than on other symptoms of grief. The drugs are the same as those used to treat depression. There is relatively little research in this area, but some studies suggest that both older-style antidepressants (known as tricyclics) and the more modern antidepressants (known as selective serotonin reuptake inhibitors: SSRIs) can be useful in lifting mood and assisting psychological therapy. Drugs that are sometimes used for short periods to overcome anxiety symptoms (benzodiazepines) have not been shown to be useful in complicated grief.

Psychological treatment for complicated grief usually involves talking through the memories of the loved one and remembering who they were and what they did. The therapy then moves on to examining the loss and what this means to the bereaved woman. This might involve visiting the grave of the deceased with the therapist. The woman needs to accept the loss and realise that, although life is inevitably different without her loved one, it can and will go on. Final stages in therapy involve helping the bereaved woman to structure and move forward in her life, while still keeping memories of her loved one.

Tips for friends and family

- In general, bereaved women do not need professional help, counselling or medication. Most women are best allowed to grieve in their own way and their own time, and in the presence of close family and friends.
- As grief is a universal experience, it can often seem to be trivialised. Following the loss of a loved one, women are often told they will 'get over it'. Whereas this is usually true, it is best not to make such comments.

- The best advice is to listen to the bereaved woman and offer support. She is not looking to you to supply answers, just support.

Useful resource

Cruse Bereavement Care
www.cruse.org.uk
08444779400
Cruse has pamphlets and self-help books that are appropriate for most situations.

References and further reading

Murray-Parkes C, Wertheimer A (2001) *A Special Scar: The Experiences of People Bereaved by Suicide* (2nd edn). Routledge.

Pringerson HG (2010) *Bereavement: Studies of Grief in Adult Life* (4th edn). Penguin.

Part IV.
Women and specific disorders

Depression and other mood disorders

Paul Blenkiron

Amanda's story

At first Amanda didn't know what was wrong. She kept waking up and worrying about her children. She stopped going shopping with her friends. She was tired all the time, and found it took a huge effort just to get dinner ready. She began to snap and shout at her family. Her husband John didn't understand what was happening and found it difficult to cope with her loss of interest in sex.

Every day Amanda felt like she was going around in a fog. She began to call in sick to work and have suicidal thoughts. John caught her with a handful of pills and convinced her to seek help. She was diagnosed with depression and prescribed antidepressant medication. Amanda began to regain her energy, appetite and ability to sleep. She also started psychological therapy, which she found helped her manage her moods and start doing normal things again. She felt the fog had lifted and was able to go back to work.

It's normal to feel sad, fed up or miserable at times. But if you feel low for weeks or months, and it's so bad it affects your life, it might be depression.

Depression is a leading cause of disability in the world today. It is very common: 1 in 5 women and 1 in 8 men are affected, often between 20 and 55 years of age. Famous women who have been depressed include the actress Angelina Jolie, the author J.K. Rowling, the singer Karen Carpenter and the comedienne Ruby Wax. The good news is that, once depression is recognised, there are effective treatments and ways to prevent it coming back.

What types of mood disorder affect women?

Clinical depression (also called major depressive disorder)

Depression is more than sadness, grief or disappointment. It can affect every area of your life, physically as well as mentally. Everyone is different, but most women with depression have at least four of the ten symptoms listed in Box 18.1.

Box 18.1 Ten symptoms of depression

D – Depressed mood (feeling low most of the time)

E – Energy lost (feeling utterly tired or irritable)

P – Pleasure lost (no interest in life, can't enjoy anything, including sex)

R – Restless (agitated) or retarded (slowed down)

E – Eating habits changed (appetite and/or weight goes up or down)

S – Sleep changed (more or less than usual)

S – Suicidal thoughts or feeling life is not worth living

I – I'm a failure (thinking you are worthless or inadequate)

O – Only me to blame (feeling guilty and self-critical)

N – No concentration (not able to function or make decisions)

Bipolar disorder (previously called manic depression)

Bipolar disorder is a serious illness that affects 1 in 50 women and men. As well as depression, there are periods of high mood lasting days to weeks. These highs are called hypomania – or mania if more severe. You feel elated, full of energy, overactive or irritable. You sleep and eat less and may behave out of character, for example, travelling, spending or making reckless plans. For some women, it can be a time when there is a real vulnerability to financial or sexual exploitation. Bipolar disorder is not the same as having quicker mood swings every few minutes or hours.

Postnatal depression

Between 10% and 30% of women become significantly depressed around the time of childbirth (Chapter 31).

Premenstrual dysphoric disorder (PMDD)

Women with PMDD feel tense, irritable, bloated and low, starting 10–14 days before menstruation. The symptoms improve after menstruation starts. Women who are prone to PMDD are also more likely to develop problems with low mood after childbirth and during the menopause.

Seasonal affective disorder (SAD)

Women with SAD get depressed in the winter when there is less daylight, but the depression goes away every spring. Symptoms include feeling tired and low, sleeping and eating more, craving carbohydrates and weight gain. It affects more women than men.

What causes depression in women?

Depression is not a sign of weakness or personal failure. You cannot just 'snap out of it'. It often runs in families, so genes are important. Life events can also trigger depression – for example, relationship difficulties, debts or losing a relative. So can drinking too much alcohol and physical health problems like arthritis, chronic pain or an underactive thyroid. In about 1 in 5 people, depression comes 'out of the blue' – that is, without an identifiable cause. Women are twice as likely as men to develop depression and there are many potential reasons for this.

- Upbringing – women are more likely to suffer from childhood trauma, sexual abuse, victimisation and domestic violence (see Chapter 7).
- Psychology – from puberty onwards, girls are more likely to worry about their body image. Women also tend more to look inwards and dwell on distressing feelings. Studies show this can trigger depression (Nolen-Hoeksema *et al*, 1999).

- Hormones – female hormones and the reproductive cycle can affect mood. This can relate to the menstrual cycle, pregnancy, childbirth, menopause, infertility, miscarriage, the contraceptive pill and hormone replacement therapy. However, it is often the life changes associated with these things rather than hormones themselves that lead to longer-lasting depression.
- Responsibilities – women are more likely to be in caring roles that make them vulnerable to depression, such as looking after small children or someone with a serious illness. When children leave home, women who have spent their lives caring for them can suffer from 'empty nest syndrome'.
- Circumstances – poverty and lack of equality or choice can affect mental health. Women make up 70% of the world's poor and two-thirds of low-paid workers and own less than 1% of the world's property (Global Citizen, 2012). A satisfying job can improve well-being, but also cause stress by clashing with childcare and home responsibilities.

Differences in depression between women and men

The symptoms and outlook for depression are similar in both genders, but there are some differences.

- Women are more likely to admit they have a problem and seek help; men frequently bottle up their feelings.
- Women report more food cravings, weight gain, fatigue and health anxiety.
- Women often 'self-medicate' using food or friends, whereas men tend to cope using distraction and activities like TV, sport or sex.
- Women tend to avoid conflict, blame themselves or criticise their appearance; men may take things out on their surroundings, get aggressive, blame others or drink heavily.

Bipolar disorder in women and men

Women with bipolar disorder are more likely than men to experience changes in their appetite and weight. They might develop an eating disorder or a thyroid problem. Women with bipolar disorder are less likely than men to have certain difficulties with their behaviour, such as over-using drugs and alcohol, gambling and trouble with the law.

In women, the menstrual cycle, pregnancy and the menopause can affect periods of depression or high mood. Women are also more likely to develop 'rapid cycling', which is having more than two episodes of highs or lows in a year. Rapid cycling often links with reproductive cycles and can mean longer, deeper depressions that can be difficult to treat. The chances of a woman developing bipolar disorder are much higher just after giving birth, but mood-stabilising medication can help to prevent this.

Treatments available

Depression often improves on its own after a few months, but there is a 50% chance it will come back in the future. Most women get help through their GP and don't need to see a psychiatrist. Treatment can involve a talking therapy, medication, or both. These work for at least 70% of women getting help via their GP. Others may need help from specialist mental health services.

Talking therapy

- Cognitive–behavioural therapy (CBT) is an effective treatment for depression and other mental health problems (Box 18.2). CBT can be done face-to-face or in groups with a professional, or at home guided by a book, mobile app or internet programme.
- Problem-solving is helpful for tackling practical problems, step by step.
- Counselling: talking through things can help (e.g. Cruse Bereavement Care).
- Couples therapy is useful for relationship problems (e.g. Relate).
- Mindfulness involves practising paying real attention to what you are doing right at this moment, rather than getting involved with upsetting thoughts.

- Interpersonal therapy and psychodynamic therapy examine how past experiences might be causing current difficulties in life and relationships.

Medication

Depression

Modern antidepressant drugs are safe and effective. They help around two-thirds of women with depression, especially in more severe cases. For many women with a mild to moderate depression, medication is not necessarily needed and other treatments are just as likely to work.

Antidepressants work by boosting levels of natural brain chemicals that can be lower in depression. Some types, such as selective serotonin reuptake inhibitors (SSRIs), might work better in women than in men. Common side-effects of SSRIs include dry mouth, headache and reduced appetite. Some people may experience dizziness, anxiety, agitation, diarrhoea, constipation or sexual problems. These usually wear off and you start noticing the benefits after 2–4 weeks.

St John's wort might also relieve mild to moderate depression, but do not take this if you take any other medication, including the contraceptive pill.

Box 18.2   What is cognitive–behavioural therapy?

Cognitive–behavioural therapy (CBT) teaches more helpful ways of thinking and reacting in everyday situations.

- Cognitive – what you think. You learn to spot when you are being negative and self-critical. You challenge thoughts such as 'I'll never get better', 'It's all going wrong' or 'I'm useless'. You develop more helpful, realistic thinking habits by asking: 'What's the evidence this is true?', 'What's another way to view this?' and 'How would I advise a friend in my situation?'
- Behavioural – what you do. You keep a daily diary of activities, then set goals to do things that boost your mood and give you a sense of achievement.
- Therapy – what you learn. CBT works best if you practise new skills as 'homework'. This helps you stay well in the future too.

Bipolar disorder

A mood-stabilising drug (e.g. lithium, valproate, quetiapine) is the main treatment for both the highs and lows of bipolar disorder, and also for prevention. Some medicines used to treat bipolar disorder can affect a fetus. It is important that women with bipolar disorder use effective contraception and discuss any plans to start a family with their GP well in advance. Valproate is best avoided in young women, as it can interfere with the reproductive system and harm the baby if the woman becomes pregnant. If a woman is taking valproate already and has been thinking about getting pregnant or falls pregnant, it is important that the GP or treating team closely monitors her health and the health of the unborn child.

Antidepressants are not usually very helpful in bipolar disorder. Women with bipolar disorder should avoid taking them on their own, as they can trigger highs or periods of overactivity and euphoria that can be difficult to control. A regular routine and plenty of sleep are also important.

Other treatments

- Some women with very severe depression, including postnatal depression, benefit from electroconvulsive therapy (ECT). This is given in a hospital under a short-acting general anaesthetic, but might not need admission to hospital overnight.
- For SAD, light-box therapy (30 min to 1 h each day) or an antidepressant are effective.
- For premenstrual syndrome, antidepressants, vitamin B6 supplements and the contraceptive pill can help.

Tips for women with a mood disorder

- Taking action can be hard, but it's worth it. Often it's the things you don't feel like doing that help.
- Recognise that you have a mood disorder. Look up your symptoms online; get professional help by talking to your general practitioner (GP) as a first step.
- Tell others how you feel – especially if you have suicidal thoughts. It does not mean you are weak or crazy.

119

- Sleep at regular times, but do not stay in bed or nap in the daytime – do something active.
- Eat regularly, with plenty of fruit and vegetables, and avoid junk food, which will only make you feel worse.
- Avoid alcohol and street drugs, as they make things worse.
- Get into a daily routine with a structure. Do the things you usually enjoy.
- Do not avoid tasks. Make a start today. Break big things into small steps.
- Exercise regularly in any way you enjoy – you could try swimming, running, yoga, going to the gym or simply walking for 15 min a day.
- Notice your negative thinking. It is like having a critical devil on your shoulder. Challenge it! Say, 'This is not me – it's the depression talking'.

Tips for family and friends

- It is not easy supporting a loved one who has depression. It's normal to feel helpless, frustrated, angry, sad or guilty.
- Support the self-help tips above for women with a mood disorder.
- Encourage her to see the family doctor. If she resists, suggest a simple check-up, and offer to go with her.
- Do not discourage her from taking medication or seeing a therapist.
- Spend time with her and listen more than talking or advising.
- Don't say 'It's all in your head', 'You've nothing to be depressed about' or 'Pull yourself together'.
- Do say 'Your depression is real', 'I'm here' and 'You may not believe it, but you will feel better'.
- Don't hide her depression, or try to rescue or 'fix' her. It is not your fault and you can't make depression 'better'.
- Take it seriously if she gets worse or talks about suicide. Make sure she tells her doctor.
- Don't take it personally if she says hurtful things.
- Take care of yourself – it is a necessity, not selfishness. You can only do so much.
- Talk to a friend or join a support group.

Staying well

Staying well depends on the three Ms: life management, mindset and medication. For women, good-quality relationships seem particularly important, whereas for men, success and achievement may protect against depression. Putting self-help approaches into practice is very useful.

For those prescribed antidepressants, it is important to continue them for 6 months or more. They are not addictive, although some women can find it hard to withdraw from them and need a very gradual reduction in dose. For repeated depression, medication can be taken safely for years (it halves the chances of the depression coming back).

Like Amanda at the start of this chapter, millions of women have overcome depression to lead happy and fulfilling lives again.

Useful resources

Bipolar UK
www.bipolaruk.org.uk
0207 931 6480

Cruse Bereavement Care
www.cruse.org.uk

Depression Alliance
www.depressionalliance.org
0845 123 2320

Depression UK
www.depressionuk.org
0870 774 4320

Free online CBT programmes for depression
www.livinglifetothefull.com
https://moodgym.anu.edu.au

Information on self-help practices
www.getselfhelp.co.uk

National Association for Premenstrual Syndrome
www.pms.org.uk
0844 815 7311

Reading Well Books on Prescription
www.reading-well.org.uk
National reading scheme that lists self-help books for depression
and other problems. Endorsed by professionals and supported
by public libraries.

Relate: The Relationship People
www.relate.org.uk
0300 100 1234

Samaritans
www.samaritans.org
08457 909090 (if suicidal or in crisis)

References and further reading

Global Citizen (2012) *Introduction to the Challenges of Achieving Gender Equality* (www.globalcitizen.org/en/content/introduction-to-the-challenges-of-achieving-gender).

Nolen-Hoeksema S, Larson J, Grayson C (1999) Explaining the gender difference in depressive symptoms. *Journal of Personality and Social Psychology*, **77**, 1061–1072.

Anxiety disorders

Lynne M. Drummond

Linda's story

Linda is a 30-year-old nurse who works part-time and has two young children. Although always an anxious person, she began noticing that she was becoming more anxious about 3 years ago. At this time her eldest child started school and she had to take her baby to nursery, drop the oldest boy at school, and then go to work at a local health centre where she worked from 10 am to 2.30 pm. She found this rushing to several places stressful and noticed she was finding it hard to concentrate because of her increasing anxiety: she was constantly worrying that she would not make it to either work or school on time.

Her husband noticed she was stressed and suggested she talk to her general practitioner (GP). Linda was reluctant at first as she felt she should be able to 'snap out of it', but eventually agreed. The GP thought that she seemed very stressed and discussed treatment options with her. Linda did not want to take medication but agreed to a referral to the local psychological well-being service for a course of cognitive–behavioural therapy (CBT). Linda's GP also encouraged her to eat regular meals, avoid excessive caffeine drinks and alcohol and stop smoking, to help reduce her symptoms. The GP told her that regular exercise also helps some women overcome some of the symptoms of anxiety.

Linda started taking good care of her general health by eating well-balanced meals, reducing her alcohol consumption to no more than a small glass of wine on a maximum of 5 days a week, reducing her coffee drinking and joining a fitness club. She went on a quit-smoking course and hasn't smoked for 6 months. Linda also attended five CBT sessions, in which the therapist helped her identify some of her 'trigger' thoughts – the ones that caused feelings of anxiety – and helped her deal with these thoughts, as well as exploring her ways of coping.

> Linda now feels well and able to enjoy life. She admits that she does become stressed and anxious at times but, instead of entering into a vicious circle of anxiety, worry and guilt, she knows she can examine the reasons she feels stressed and try to work out the best possible solutions.

Every woman experiences anxiety at times in her life. In fact, if we were unable to experience fear and anxiety it would be very dangerous, as we would go into dangerous situations without thinking of the consequences. In addition, there are optimal levels of anxiety that help us to perform tasks. For example, a driver who has a healthy respect for the potential danger of the roads is likely to be a safer and better driver than someone who is overly confident (or very anxious).

The idea of 'clinical' or 'pathological' anxiety is a relative term. In other words, the anxiety is simply more frequent or more intense than the person can tolerate. Women have traditionally been more willing to admit to anxiety, whereas men have been encouraged to hide their fears. Anxiety disorders include specific fears, which are called phobias, and more general fears in the form of generalised anxiety disorder and panic disorder.

Phobia

A phobia is an irrational fear of a situation or object that most people would consider non-threatening. Everyone has some irrational fears and dislikes, but a true phobia causes distress and interferes with normal day-to-day living.

Many phobias start in childhood or adolescence and can continue into adulthood. The phobias children have include fears of specific animals (e.g. dogs, cats, spiders), of social situations or performing certain acts such as eating or drinking in public, and of medical or dental procedures and the sight of blood (known as blood and injury phobia). There are many other specific phobias, such as fears of thunder, heights or flying. One phobia that only occurs in children is school phobia or school refusal. This is quite common in anxious children, and while most fully recover, a few go on to develop agoraphobia or other anxiety problems later.

The most common phobia is agoraphobia. A woman with agoraphobia is anxious in crowded places such as public transport, busy supermarkets and places where she feels she cannot escape. Agoraphobia and specific animal phobias are more common in women than men, but social phobia, blood and injury phobia and miscellaneous specific phobias occur equally in women and men. Agoraphobia usually starts in the 20s.

Generalised anxiety disorder

Generalised anxiety disorder refers to a more general experience of anxiety. All of us vary in the amount and intensity of anxiety we feel. Generalised anxiety disorder is diagnosed when there is a troublesome increase in anxiety that interferes with a person getting on with her life. The widespread anxiety and worrying can be debilitating.

Generalised anxiety disorder is more common in women than men. It can also be part of a depressive illness.

Panic disorder

In this condition, the person experiences extreme bouts of anxiety that often seem to come out of the blue. These bouts are accompanied by physical symptoms:

- difficulty breathing
- palpitations and feeling that the heart is beating too fast
- pins and needles in the fingers and toes
- a sense of impending death or that something terrible is going to happen.

These bouts sometimes happen in the middle of the night. Because these sorts of symptoms occur in some physical illnesses, many women have multiple medical tests before the diagnosis of panic disorder is made. These investigations are important but can, in themselves, raise anxiety. Panic disorder can occur alone or with agoraphobia and other anxiety disorders. Women are twice as likely as men to suffer from panic disorder.

Treatment

Cognitive–behavioural therapy (CBT) is the main psychological treatment for anxiety disorders. The therapeutic approach used will depend on the nature of the specific problem.

CBT for phobia

For a phobic disorder, the woman and her therapist will work out a hierarchy of fear-provoking situations and, with the help of her therapist, the woman learns how to face these situations in a systematic manner. She will need to practise homework exercises regularly (at least twice a day) and for long enough each time for the anxiety to subside (usually an hour, at least initially). Once she has achieved the first steps on the hierarchy, the woman can move on to more difficult items until she covers the whole hierarchy. This treatment works for almost all women with phobias.

CBT for generalised anxiety disorder

For generalised anxiety disorder, CBT generally involves the woman and her therapist examining the thoughts that tend to precede anxiety episodes and piecing together evidence for or against these thoughts. The therapist will also give the woman practical exercises and assistance to overcome the symptoms of generalised anxiety.

CBT for panic disorder

For panic disorder, CBT might specifically focus on the catastrophic thoughts that women with this disorder often have. For example, the woman may notice her heart is beating faster than normal and might think, 'My heart is beating so fast, it will stop and I will die'. Having that thought will increase her anxiety and worsen her symptoms, reinforcing her belief that she might die. Therapy needs to break this connection using education and a number of practical experiments and tests, which the woman and her therapist can construct together.

Medication

Sometimes a selective serotonin reuptake inhibitor (SSRI) is useful in the treatment of an anxiety disorder. These drugs are not addictive and the woman will need to take the SSRI regularly for some months (and sometimes longer); they are not effective if the woman only takes them when she feels as though she needs extra help. It is best to gradually reduce and stop this medication with support from a GP to reduce the chance of any relapse.

Pitfalls to avoid are the use of alcohol to give 'Dutch courage' and the use of tranquilisers, including benzodiazepine drugs such as diazepam (Valium). These drugs are addictive, so their use can lead to reliance and a need to increase the dose to get the same effect. Benzodiazepines should only ever be taken for less than 6 weeks at a time, and only under medical supervision.

Tips for family and friends

- Avoid judgement: a woman cannot 'snap out of' anxiety disorders and she is not being 'silly' or 'melodramatic'.
- It is important to encourage the woman to visit her GP. There are psychological therapy services in the community that the GP can help the woman to access for treatment.

Useful resources

Anxiety UK
www.anxietyuk.org.uk
A self-help organisation that aims to offer support for those suffering from anxiety disorders.

NHS Choices
www.nhs.uk/conditions/anxiety
Information about anxiety disorders.

Triumph over Phobia (TOP UK)
www.topuk.org
A self-help organisation offering self-help treatment groups for people suffering from phobia and OCD.

References and furhter reading

Eastham C (2016) *We're All Mad Here: The No-Nonsense Guide to Living with Social Anxiety*. Jessica Kingsley Publishers.

Marks IM (2001) *Living with Fear: Understanding and Coping with Anxiety* (2nd edn). McGraw–Hill.

Trauma and post-traumatic stress disorder

Nuri Gené-Cos

Razia's story

Razia, a shy and frightened Somalian woman, came to my clinic complaining of headaches. Since an operation several months before, her problems had got worse. Since the birth of her 7-year-old boy, Razia had been unable to sit down for any length of time owing to marked discomfort in the pelvic floor area. With little understanding of Razia's difficulties, her gynaecologist had tried to address her severe discomfort by operating on an episiotomy scar.

A female interpreter was present during the interview, but Razia refused to allow her husband in the room. She informed us of the following: she had fled her home country with her husband and her two children 10 years ago owing to the war situation. A week before her departure, she had been gang-raped in front of her children: her 3-year-old daughter was held by one of the soldiers in front of her while the rape took place; the 18-month-old toddler was around crying. She never told her husband, who at the time was serving on the front line. 'We were alive', she said. 'I washed myself and carried on as if it hadn't happened. If I had told him, he would be obliged to take revenge and he could be killed.'

After a dangerous journey, they got to the UK. Social Services and other people helped them. They obtained refugee status after an amnesty. Razia became pregnant and, after the birth of her second son, she developed severe symptoms of anxiety – nightmares, flashbacks and panic attacks. In addition, she became unable to sit down as this would trigger flashbacks and intrusive thoughts of the rape. She underwent trauma therapy, but did not respond to treatment. She spent the next 7 years in bed, more and more disabled by her symptoms and unable to look after her family; her husband became the main carer.

Razia understood some English but her ability to concentrate was poor and her fears made it impossible for her to go to classes, or relate to her neighbours or people from her country. She was determined to get better, as 'My children need me', but did not know how to go ahead. She was almost illiterate, having had limited access to education while growing up. Her husband was better educated and owned his own land and livestock.

Razia underwent 18 months of trauma therapy. The process was painful but she showed determination and courage. 'My children need me and you are a wise woman, I know I will get better.'

Towards the end of the treatment, Razia complained that her younger son, by now 9 years old, had severe reading difficulties. She wanted to help him but felt helpless, so we addressed this in therapy. Razia decided to meet with her son's school headmaster, and it was agreed to provide him with a tutor. She came back radiant, saying 'I got the tutor, my boy will be fine'. That day, we both knew that she had made it. The worst part of her trauma had been knowing that she was unable to protect her children, but this time she had managed it.

Four years later, I was on my lunch break in the canteen when a slim, uniformed woman came towards me and hugged me. Razia spoke in English and she had come to tell me that she was starting a restaurant job that day. 'I want you to see me dressed in my uniform, to thank you,' she said warmly. We held hands. She mentioned that her husband was also working and the children were doing well. In one of my shopping trips to the city centre, I decided to visit the restaurant where Razia worked; I saw her sitting in a relaxed way and smiling at a client, a remembrance poppy in her uniform cap. As I was leaving without – I thought – her noticing me, she turned towards me and said, 'Bye sweetheart'.

Women and migration

Immigration implies planning and some flexibility in the choice of country. However, for immigrants in extreme poverty, or for refugees/asylum seekers, the sense of having a choice is often missing. Although immigrants may have experienced duress, asylum seekers by definition come from war or other intense social conflicts, where they have often endured life-threatening situations and witnessed the deaths of family members. They leave behind most of their possessions as well as loved ones.

Post-traumatic stress disorder

Edith's story

Edith sat in my office, dressed in black, looking many years younger than her 48 years of age. She had been raped, in a date rape, 5 years earlier and since then, although able to maintain a job as a graphic designer in a big company, she had struggled to cope in many areas of her life. She had given up on everything except paying her bills. Since the rape, she had lost the sense of her capabilities: 'I was planning to go solo ... then that happened ... I have never dared to do much'.

Edith reported dissociative symptoms (mainly numbing herself and disconnecting from her surroundings) as well as hyperarousal symptoms (severe anxiety, becoming panicked easily, irritable without apparent reason and paranoid when people walked close to her in the street, particularly men). She was easily startled by minor noises even when in her own home. In addition, she often had nightmares and flashbacks of the rape.

Over the 5 years following the rape, Edith had developed a series of coping strategies, including self-harming, avoiding specific areas of the city she lived in and constantly screening for 'a particular type of man'. She was hypervigilant most of the time and would frequently wake up at night. She told her family about the rape, and their negative response to her not being able to cope with the trauma made her feel increasingly isolated and 'let down'.

Edith got married in her late 20s and divorced 15 years later. She decided to join a dating agency. On the day of the rape, she went out with a man. 'The guy wasn't my type, I knew it from the beginning, but I thought let's have dinner, a chat and goodbye.' She could hardly remember what they had eaten or what their conversation had been. Her senses muddled up smells, colours and fragments of conversations. The next thing she was aware of was being at home with him. 'He was hurting me and I could not defend myself,' she said. She reported the rape, but 'the police did not believe me'. This added a sense of moral injury to the assault. She felt bitter and deeply betrayed that she could not get 'justice for what happened'.

We started therapy soon after the initial assessment. Edith had tried several therapies, but did not find them helpful, so she was sceptical as to what to expect. She found the new therapy (sensorimotor psychotherapy) challenging, so we slowed down the process while she learned to develop new strategies to cope with her symptoms without needing to avoid or dissociate as much. We agreed to interweave lifespan integration therapy with sensorimotor psychotherapy.

Lifespan integration therapy is a new approach that promotes healing by integrating fragmented memories of experiences into a 'life movie' that allows the woman to move on.

Edith also had severe depression and anxiety and the strain of therapy was causing her already run-down energy levels and coping mechanisms to flounder. She began to take antidepressant medication.

During the early therapy sessions, Edith would panic easily and then feel defeated by the feeling that she would never get better. 'I have been like this for so long,' she said. After several months, Edith noticed that she was able to manage better while at work and able to regulate her fears more easily while in the street. It took almost a year of therapy for Edith to be able to work directly with trauma memories.

Eventually, Edith was well enough to be discharged from the clinic. By then, she had begun writing a blog to help other victims of similar events. In her blog, she would talk about her trauma experience as well as what she was finding helpful for her recovery. She went on to set up as an independent designer.

Edith contacted me a year after her discharge. She mentioned how elated she had been after she ended therapy and felt free from her 'terrors'. 'I had a sense that I could do anything ... I was high. I could not believe I could feel normal, I was in touch with my ambitions.' However, she was able to understand her mood changes and to feel that the present belonged to her and her alone.

After a traumatic event, women may develop stress symptoms that later subside. But for a number of women this is not the case, and they go on to develop post-traumatic stress disorder (PTSD). Although the reasons are unclear, women are more susceptible than men to developing PTSD. Factors such as the difference in physical strength between victim and perpetrator, as well as specific types of violence, such as rape, may explain the difference.

Symptoms

The main symptoms of PTSD are reliving the traumatic events via flashbacks and nightmares and, when reminded of the trauma, physical and emotional symptoms. The woman avoids anything that triggers memories of the trauma. She might feel numb and be unable to feel close to loved ones. She can become suspicious, irritable and hypersensitive to noises. She may also suffer insomnia and poor concentration.

Treatment

If PTSD is left untreated, it often becomes chronic; this will have a serious impact on the woman and her personal or family life. When a woman is the main carer of her children, it is important to treat her condition as soon as possible to avoid damage to the children. Research has also shown that, with mothers suffering from PTSD at the time of pregnancy or soon after giving birth, their children may develop a vulnerability to similar problems.

How we understand trauma varies from one culture to another; the attitude to rape and sexual exploitation is a major source of shame in many cultures and may block the treatment, as well as producing social isolation. In some cultures there is no specific concept of trauma, and so the woman may not express herself in psychological terms but with physical symptoms; this may be more common in women than men.

There is a range of talking therapies for PTSD.

- Cognitive–behavioural therapy (CBT): a talking treatment which can help us to understand how 'habits of thinking' can make the PTSD worse – or even cause it. CBT can help you change these 'extreme' ways of thinking, which can help you to feel better and to behave differently.
- Eye-movement desensitisation and reprocessing (EMDR): a technique that uses eye movements to help the brain to process flashbacks and to make sense of the traumatic experience. It may sound odd, but it can work well.
- Sensorimotor psychotherapy: a body-centred therapy to relieve the devastating effects of trauma. It is a way of listening to sensations within the body and becoming more aware, so that feelings and memories can come to the surface.

In the case of refugees, the therapist will have to adjust to the individual's cultural understanding in order to address their symptoms. Medication may be useful when there is marked insomnia, depression or symptoms of psychosis, as well as when a woman is not able to undergo therapy. Psychoeducation helps the woman and her family or carers to deal with her condition in the best way possible.

The process of changing country and ongoing legal procedures, as well as social discrimination, will often have a major impact on a woman's personal/family life. If one member of the family suffers from PTSD, it is important to screen other members for related conditions.

Tips for family and friends

- Try to understand how PTSD may affect the woman's behaviour and try not to judge.
- Contact support organisations or self-help groups.
- Support the woman in practical issues and encourage a normal routine as much as possible.
- Look out for changes in behaviour that may lead to the woman not coping and try to learn what the main triggers are.
- Be patient: recovery may take some time.

Useful resources

British Red Cross
www.redcross.org.uk
The Red Cross can help find missing relatives. Their services are free and confidential.

Freedom From Torture
www.freedomfromtorture.org
Provides support and counselling for survivors of torture in the UK.

Human Rights Watch
www.hrw.org
A non-profit human rights organisation that publishes reports and briefings on human rights conditions in 90 countries.

Refugee Action
www.refugeeaction.org.uk
Provides advice and practical support for refugees and asylum seekers.

Refugee Council
www.refugeecouncil.org.uk
An organisation that works with refugees and people seeking asylum in the UK.

RefugeeMap

Refugeemap.wikidot.com

Information on refugee situations, news, policy and volunteering.

References and further reading

Herman J (2015) *Trauma and Recovery. The Aftermath of Violence – From Domestic Abuse to Political Terror.* Basic Books.

Yehuda R, Engel SM, Brand SR, *et al* (2005) Transgenerational effects of post-traumatic stress disorder in babies of mothers exposed to the World Trade Centre attack during pregnancy. *Journal of Clinical Endocrinology and Metabolism,* **90,** 4115–4118.

World Health Organization (2013) *Guidelines for the Management of Conditions Specifically Related to Stress.* WHO.

The dangers of rumination

Raj Persaud

Kim's story (part 1)

Kim had never really recovered from the upset of finding a breast lump. Her mother had died of breast cancer in her mid-40s, so the discovery of the lump brought back memories from the darkest period in her life, although the lump was eventually diagnosed as benign. Kim panicked that she did indeed have cancer herself. She subsequently became preoccupied with whether to find out if she carried the breast cancer gene. If her genetic risk was high enough, she might consider a preventive mastectomy.

Kim spent all her time at work searching the internet for information on genetics and breast cancer, leading her into trouble with her boss. On top of that, her boyfriend was becoming exasperated by the fact she could discuss nothing but tumour research and the latest celebrity to be diagnosed with cancer. A surgeon she consulted tried to explain that she needed to stop obsessing about breast cancer. But this only seemed to make things worse. Kim became convinced she must be going mad, because she realised she was unable to control her own thoughts and cease brooding.

Women are twice as likely as men to have serious feelings of depression. Some forms of low mood are very specific to women, including the 'baby blues', postpartum depression, sadness around menopause, and melancholy linked to menstruation. However, the gap between rates of severe depressive feelings in women and men has been narrowing in recent years. Improved access to education, employment and effective birth control might have reduced women's exposure to stress. Women today have more access to what might have traditionally helped men deal with negative feelings – the distraction of work outside the home, a wider social circle (with office colleagues) and financial independence.

Surveys have found that women tend to report more positive emotions as well as more negative ones (Fujita *et al*, 1991). Women might experience more emotion, or more variation in emotion, or they might simply be more aware of their moods than men are.

Studies suggest women have more 'internalising' disorders, in which difficulties centre on an unpleasant internal experience (e.g. depression, anxiety, panic, phobia). Men tend to have more 'externalising' disorders, in which outward behaviour is problematic (e.g. attention-deficit hyperactivity disorder, violence, alcohol and drug dependency) (Kramer *et al*, 2008).

Another way of understanding this difference is that women tend to brood and ruminate more than men. Rumination involves repetitive, negative and intrusive thoughts, usually focusing on distress. This can make low mood and anxiety worse by dwelling too much on problems, making them seem unsolvable.

Susan Nolen-Hoeksema (1991), a world authority on the subject, defines rumination as a passive focus on symptoms of distress and on all the possible causes and consequences. An example is sitting alone and dwelling on how tired and unmotivated you feel, and then worrying that your mood will interfere with your job, career and life.

Nolen-Hoeksema & Jackson (2001) found that women were more likely than men to believe they should focus on their emotions rather than taking action (problem-solving), were more likely to be convinced that negative moods and what causes them are uncontrollable, and furthermore were more likely to feel responsible for the emotional tone of their relationships. These beliefs mean women tend to focus intently on their own emotions, particularly negative ones; leading them to be wary of taking actions to tackle sources of distress; and, so, to engage in more rumination than men.

Rumination can get in the way of helpful action when confronted with a problem. For example, when asked to anticipate their reaction to discovering a breast lump, researchers found that 'ruminators' were less likely to report seeking a medical consultation. Among breast cancer survivors, ruminators delayed reporting initial cancer symptoms to a doctor by a margin of 2 months compared with non-ruminators (Lyubomirsky *et al*, 2006). Ruminators are also more likely to experience excessive dependency and neediness in relationships and assume too much responsibility for the well-being of others.

The best way to combat a tendency to ruminate is to not focus on the issues that preoccupy. Of course, asking ruminators simply to stop obsessing about their worry is rarely helpful. It can even make some people feel worse in the short term. Pleasant distractions, such as watching an interesting film or playing a favourite sport, are more effective at improving mood and reducing brooding. But rumination itself reduces the motivation to engage in such distracting activities, so scheduling them into a planned timetable can be necessary.

Mindfulness exercises, borrowed from meditation and relaxation techniques, involve distancing yourself from your thoughts. The idea is to recognise that you are separate from your thoughts. These exercises are also useful in a number of anxiety-related disorders.

Kim's story (part 2)

After Kim watched a favourite movie as 'homework', she was asked to report her observations. She noticed that when distracted for a while from her worries, she felt a little better. She also saw that dwelling on breast cancer (whether before or after the movie) made no difference to her plan, which was to postpone any decision until she had seen a genetic counsellor. Kim realised that watching the film focused her attention elsewhere, and that this helped her mood. She understood she could become better at directing her attention.

Kim was encouraged to become aware that there are different ways of thinking about a problem. An alternative to rumination is to seek an action plan. If no practical action was possible, then she could at least begin to see that ruminating was not productive. She scheduled time into her day when she was allowed to worry – half an hour after lunch. Outside that time, she was to distract herself by doing interesting work or focusing on her relationship. When she found herself ruminating, she changed tack and came up with some kind of action plan.

Kim found she was better able to keep her worry in check until she finally got to see the genetic counsellor, whose advice was that a mastectomy was unnecessary. She could now better take the 'helicopter' position, a term used in therapy about being able to look down on yourself, gaining more perspective. Just being able to label her inner life with terms such as 'worry' and 'rumination' had helped her distance herself from painful feelings.

References and further reading

Fujita F, Diener E, Sandvik E (1991) Gender differences in negative affect and well-being: the case for emotional intensity. *Journal of Personality and Social Psychology*, **61**, 427–434.

Kramer MD, Krueger RF, Hicks BM (2008) The role of internalizing and externalizing liability factors in accounting for gender differences in the prevalence of common psychopathological syndromes. *Psychological Medicine*, **38**, 51–61.

Lyubomirsky S, Kasri F, Chang O, *et al* (2006) Ruminative response styles and delay of seeking diagnosis for breast cancer symptoms. *Journal of Social and Clinical Psychology*, **25**, 276–304.

Nolen-Hoeksema S (1991) Responses to depression and their effects on the duration of depressive episodes. *Journal of Abnormal Psychology*, **100**, 569–582.

Nolen-Hoeksema S, Jackson B (2001) Mediators of the gender difference in rumination. *Psychology of Women Quarterly*, **25**, 37–47.

Obsessive–compulsive disorder

Lynne M. Drummond

Marina's story

Marina is a 30-year-old married woman with two young children. A few years ago, her youngest son, George, became seriously ill with meningitis. Although George recovered well, Marina started to worry about her children catching serious illnesses and dying. She began to clean the house meticulously, scrubbing the entire kitchen and bathroom with bleach every day. If she touched anything touched by non-family members, she would wash her hands, and she constantly used antiseptic hand gel. Her hand-washing increased until she was doing it almost 100 times a day. Bathing or showering could take up to 3h, as she felt the urge to wash until she felt certain she was completely clean. As a result, her hands became chapped and she developed bodily eczema. The children were discouraged from mixing with friends apart from at school, and Marina told them to use antiseptic hand gel at all times. When they returned from school, they had to take off all their clothes in the hallway; Marina washed the clothes immediately, while the children had a bath. Marina's husband had become so concerned about her vigorous washing of the children that he had started returning home at the end of the school day to supervise more 'normal' washing of the children, before he then returned to his work as an electrician.

Every attempt by her husband and mother to encourage Marina to seek help had failed. She felt too embarrassed to own up to the problem and felt she was doing her best to keep the children well and happy. After a discussion with her mother, Marina began to realise that her children were living a very restricted life and that they should have more freedom. She also worried that Social Services might become involved in the family and so, reluctantly, went to her general practitioner (GP).

Marina's GP talked to her about treatments for obsessive–compulsive disorder (OCD). Initially, she had the choice of starting on a medication and psychological treatment involving graded exposure. Marina felt she would prefer to try a psychological approach first, and her GP referred her to the local psychological therapy service.

The sessions were hard work. Marina would form a list of 'exposure tasks' to perform without 'undoing' her actions by washing or cleaning. Marina and the therapist graded the exposure tasks from the easiest (touching a door handle outside the house without washing her hands or using gel) to the most difficult (allowing the children to have friends round to play in the house without Marina 'decontaminating' every area they touched). Every week, she would perform an exposure task with her therapist; her homework was to practise this task three times a day at home before the next session. Progress was slow and Marina continued to see the therapist for 20 sessions over the next 5 months. She gradually began to make improvements and her husband remarked how much happier and more outgoing the children had become as Marina progressed.

After therapy ended, Marina felt confident she had skills to continue to improve. She realised that everyone has good and bad times, and that she would always have a tendency, at times of stress, to develop symptoms. However, she now felt confident that she could cope with any obsessive thoughts and not give into compulsions so that the disorder did not take control of her life again.

Obsessive–compulsive disorder

OCD will affect about 2% of women over their lifetime. The severity of the disorder varies from mild (causing minor inconvenience) to very serious (when every aspect of a woman's life changes and her physical health and well-being are significantly impaired).

OCD is equally common in women and men and usually starts in childhood or early adult life. If it is picked up in childhood, most children respond well to treatment, but in a few the disorder continues into adulthood.

OCD includes obsessions and compulsions. Although we talk lightly about people being 'obsessed', OCD obsessions are very different. They are horrible, worrying and persistent thoughts, images or impulses which come into the person's mind and cause extreme distress. For example, thoughts that germs from other people will cause harm to them or their family, images of themselves stabbing a much-loved family member or the impulse to attack strangers in the street. These thoughts, images or impulses are abhorrent to the individual, who will take extreme precautions to prevent them coming true or avoid acting on them. A woman with an obsessive fear that she may sexually molest children finds this thought offensive, and will go to great lengths to ensure it does not happen. This is important as healthcare professionals will be concerned if someone says she is frightened that she may molest children. However, people with OCD are unlikely to act on such thoughts.

Compulsions are acts, thoughts or images designed to reduce or prevent the anxiety and 'harm' from the obsessive thoughts. Examples include a mother who is frightened of dirt and germs from toilets causing her and her family illness and as a result she spends hours every day scrubbing the kitchen and toilet with bleach, and many hours in the shower ensuring she is 'clean' and 'uncontaminated'; or a daughter with visions of herself losing control and stabbing her parents to death spending all her time ensuring that any knives or potentially sharp objects are out of her reach and praying for hours a day that she would not kill her parents in this way.

Compulsions may reduce the anxiety caused by obsessive thoughts, but they are inefficient and tend to only work for a short time. For this reason, people with OCD will repeat their compulsive behaviours many times. In extreme cases, the person's life becomes consumed by OCD activity – to the point that they neglect self-care, and fail to eat and drink properly.

Treatments

Despite the serious nature of some types of OCD, it responds well to treatment. There are two main approaches.

Cognitive–behavioural therapy (CBT)

The type of CBT used in OCD is known as graded exposure. The therapist asks the patient to devise a hierarchy of fear-provoking situations and helps her to face up to these in a systematic manner, without performing compulsions. The patient needs to perform these exercises regularly (at least twice a day) and for sufficient time for the anxiety to subside (at least an hour initially). Once the patient has mastered the first steps on the hierarchy, she can move on to more difficult items until she has covered the whole hierarchy. This treatment is very effective for most women with OCD, and as many as 8 out of 10 will improve greatly if they stick with the treatment.

Selective serotonin-reuptake inhibitors (SSRIs)

SSRIs are a class of drugs that act on the serotonin pathways in the brain. They're often used as antidepressants. A higher dose is used for OCD than for depression. The drugs are not addictive, but women with OCD will need to take them for many months, or sometimes throughout their life, because for some there is a chance of relapse if they stop the treatment. There are many SSRIs and different people respond differently to the various SSRIs, so even if one drug does not help, changing to another may be the answer. Approximately 60% of people with OCD who are prescribed an SSRI will improve.

Dopamine blockers

A few people do not respond to CBT or SSRIs. However, they might respond to drugs known as dopamine blockers. These are used for psychotic conditions, but for OCD a lower dose of the drug is used (this means there is a smaller chance of side-effects).

Specialist treatment centres

Some people do not recover even with the above treatments and need to get help at a specialised treatment centre.

Related conditions

Other, similar conditions are included in the classification of OCD.

- Body dysmorphic disorder (see Chapter 23) occurs when an individual is preoccupied by imagined or greatly exaggerated defects in their appearance.
- Hoarding disorder occurs when someone forms a close attachment to objects and lives in a state of inconvenience and even squalor due to the number of their possessions.

- Trichotillomania, or compulsive hair-pulling and skin-picking disorder, is when the hair or skin is compulsively picked and damaged.

All these conditions can occur alone or in combination with OCD. The approach to treatment is similar to that for OCD.

Tips for women with OCD

If you feel you have obsessions and compulsions, it is possible to help yourself. The first thing is to identify your obsessions or the intrusive worrying thoughts that come into your head. Second, identify your compulsions – that is, any behaviours, thoughts or reassurance-seeking that you do to reduce the fear and discomfort you feel when having the obsessive thoughts. You need to stop these compulsions. People often try to cut down on compulsions, but this is not really helpful: it's much easier to entirely stop a habitual behaviour and replace it with a new, healthy behaviour than it is to cut down.

For example, if you are washing your hands repeatedly and for a prolonged time, it is easier to stop this completely than try to reduce the frequency or duration. Instead, introduce a new, short hand-washing routine before handling food and after using the toilet. In this case, you should place the plug in the sink rather than having flowing water. You can then wash your hands to below the wrist for the duration it takes to sing *Happy Birthday* twice in your head (approximately 20–30 s).

Next, identify situations, places and activities that you're avoiding to reduce your obsessive thoughts. Write these down and score how anxiety- or discomfort-provoking it would be to face up to them. Use a scale of 0–8:

- 0 = no discomfort
- 2 = mild discomfort
- 4 = moderate discomfort
- 6 = severe discomfort
- 8 = the most discomfort it is possible to feel.

Now identify a situation that would cause you mild to moderate discomfort if you faced up to it without your compulsions. Set yourself the task of facing this fear three times a day without compulsions. It can take up to 2 h for your anxiety or discomfort to fully abate, but it will get better if you stick with it. The more frequently you can carry out this exposure task, the easier it will become. Once you have conquered this task, move on to another.

Some people will find this self-help programme too difficult without outside help. You can obtain help from a self-help book, a self-help treatment group (such as those run by Triumph over Phobia UK), or a therapist. In some cases, the necessary help might be medication.

Tips for families and friends

When a loved one is distressed by OCD, it is tempting to try and relieve her suffering by helping her perform compulsions, giving endless reassurance and taking over tasks that she wishes to avoid. Although this is a normal, caring reaction, it does not help and can worsen the situation.

It is better to try and discuss how her fears seem to relate to OCD and encourage her to seek help from a GP, who can refer her to a local psychological therapy service. If psychological therapy is unsuccessful, more specialised help might be necessary via the local mental health service. If the disorder is very difficult to treat, there are highly specialised services available for OCD and related disorders.

Occasionally, someone with OCD can become insistent and bullying if you do not comply with their rules and compulsions. You should never place yourself in a situation of potential harm to yourself. If you feel threatened by a loved one, you should call the police, just as you would in any other threatening situation.

Useful resources

OCD Action
www.ocdaction.org.uk
Support network, information and telephone advice for OCD, hoarding and related disorders. Support for young people and adults of all ages.

OCD UK
www.ocduk.org
Support network, information and telephone advice for OCD and related disorders.

Triumph over Phobia (TOP UK)
www.topuk.org
A self-help organisation offering self-help treatment groups for
people with phobia and/or OCD.

References and further reading

Marks IM (2001) *Living With Fear: Understanding And Coping With Anxiety* (2nd edn). McGraw–Hill.

Stein DS, Fineberg NA (2007) *Obsessive–Compulsive Disorder*. Oxford University Press.

Eating disorders and body dysmorphic disorder

Sandeep Ranote, Andrea Phillipou, Susan Rossell and David Castle[†]

'Who wants to recover? It took me years to get that tiny. I wasn't sick; I was strong.'
– Laurie Halse Anderson (2011)

Jo's story

Looking back, I didn't think I was ill at the start. I felt in control and I felt good because I was thin, which made me feel strong and successful. Aren't all successful women thin and beautiful?

That was when I was 15 years old; at 19, I know that none of that is true. I did have an illness, a real illness that hit me in secondary school, preparing for important exams while also breaking up with my first boyfriend.

I thought I wasn't beautiful enough for him and the break-up meant that I also lost my peer group at the time. I felt alone, under pressure and hated myself. I started to diet, like most people do, and joined the gym. I started getting results, which for me was important, in the same way exams were. I lost weight and saw this as positive, so I began to do more exercise, eat less and stopped eating sugary and fatty foods. I didn't see my headaches and dizziness as a problem, I just thought I needed to sleep more. But eventually I wasn't sleeping and my grades began to drop. I felt tired and low and remember sometimes having thoughts that I no longer wanted to live.

I didn't understand why my parents were anxious and arguing with each other about me. They could see something was wrong but I couldn't see it; they tried to talk to me but I couldn't hear them. When I fainted, I was taken to hospital, and this was when I accepted and started treatment with a

---

[†]Sandeep Ranote is the author of the eating disorders section of this chapter. Andrea Phillipou, Susan Rossell and David Castle are the authors of the body dysmorphic disorder section of this chapter.

specialist eating disorder team, who became almost part of our family. They gave not only me much needed support but also the whole family.

My message to you all is that there is hope and you can get help. Don't delay, share your concerns, get the treatment and don't let this illness steal your life.

Eating disorders

Self-starvation in women is not a modern phenomenon. Medieval women in the 13th century believed it would lead to sainthood, sometimes referred to as 'anorexia mirabilis'. Sir William Gull, doctor to Queen Victoria, and Ernest-Charles Lasègue, a physician at the Salpêtrière Hospital in Paris, wrote the first medical accounts of anorexia nervosa in 1873. Until the latter part of the 20th century, public awareness of and research into eating disorders were limited. The disorders were thought to affect only wealthy, White, Western women.

We now know this is not the case. Eating disorders are complex illnesses involving psychological, social and neurobiological factors. They affect women from all cultural backgrounds and, although ten times more common in women, can also affect men. They are chronic, often long-term, life-threatening illnesses like diabetes, yet the stigma that still attaches to them is powerful and often the reason that women suffer in silence.

The most common eating disorders in the UK are anorexia nervosa and bulimia nervosa, and it is common to have both anorexia and bulimia at different times. In the UK, about 1 in every 150 teenage girls has anorexia. It often begins in adolescence and is the most life-threatening mental illness in young women. Anorexia is becoming more common in primary school children and also in girls of South Asian ethnicity born in the UK. About 1 in 250 females and 1 in 2000 males will experience anorexia nervosa in adolescence and young adulthood, and three times that number will suffer from bulimia nervosa (Beat, 2015; NHS Choices, 2015). Bulimia can also start in the teenage years, but it tends to be more noticeable in the 20s, as this is an eating disorder that can remain hidden for some time. The various signs and symptoms of anorexia and bulimia are listed in Box 23.1.

Box 23.1 Signs and symptoms of anorexia and bulimia

Anorexia

- Eating less, preoccupation with weight loss
- Fear of weight gain
- Excessive exercise
- Use of laxatives, slimming pills, amphetamines or herbal remedies to lose weight
- Calorie counting, checking weight
- Distorted view of body
- Occasional bingeing
- Social withdrawal
- Loss of interest in sex
- Monthly menstrual periods become irregular or stop
- Low mood, difficulty sleeping and concentrating
- Depressive illness, anxiety and obsessive–compulsive illnesses can develop
- Physical symptoms:
  - problems with hair, skin and nails
  - feeling cold
  - cramps, constipation and diarrhoea
  - headaches
  - dizziness
  - tiredness
  - chest pain
  - brittle bones
  - fertility problems

Bulimia

- Worrying about weight and shape
- Pattern of binge eating followed by self-induced vomiting, laxative use, excessive exercise or dieting
- Monthly menstrual periods become irregular or stop
- Feeling tired and guilty
- Staying normal weight or above in spite of dieting
- Low mood and often depressive illness
- Physical symptoms:
  - abdominal cramps
  - problems with teeth due to vomiting
  - fertility problems

Causes of eating disorders

Much has been blamed on the media, fashion industry and celebrity influences, and certainly these factors do contribute, but there is no concrete evidence that they are a primary cause of eating disorders. Certainly there were no celebrity magazines in medieval or Victorian England.

Eating disorders usually have multiple causes, which might include:

- sensitive or perfectionist personality traits
- genetics (a family history, which may not always be known)
- emotional distress
- puberty
- bullying.

New research suggests that the brains of women with eating disorders might function differently and therefore respond to stimuli differently from the brains of healthy women (Rosen, 2013). It isn't yet clear whether these differences are a cause or an effect of the illness.

Treatment

The National Institute for Health and Care Excellence (NICE, 2004) developed the first set of national guidelines for the treatment of eating disorders. Since then, national guidelines for developing eating disorder services have been published, as well as important guidelines on how to treat severely unwell women and adolescents with anorexia (Royal College of Psychiatrists, 2012, 2014). This has helped more specialist services to grow.

For every woman with an eating disorder, it is vital that her individual circumstances and support networks are understood and that a personalised programme of care is developed in partnership with her. This enables the woman's needs to be met as a whole person, not solely as a patient with anorexia or bulimia. Supporting women to share their recovery stories with others can be extremely helpful. A combination of illness education, individual therapy, diet and nutrition support, psychiatric and medical support, and family therapy makes the most successful treatment. If the woman also has a depressive disorder, anxiety or obsessive–compulsive disorder, medication can be helpful.

No one type of treatment works better than another for anorexia. Common therapies are cognitive–behavioural therapy (CBT), a motivational approach and creative therapies. Family therapy is particularly important when working with adolescent girls. For bulimia, CBT combined with selective serotonin reuptake inhibitor (SSRI) medication can improve symptoms and promote recovery.

With treatment, 60–70% of women with anorexia or bulimia will recover, or at least improve. In one study of people with anorexia, 46% made a full recovery, 33% improved without making a full recovery and 20% remained chronically ill. A study of people with bulimia found that 45% recovered, 27% significantly improved and 23% remained chronically ill (Beat, 2015).

Research, particularly using brain imaging, is ever-continuing so that more effective treatments can be developed: medications, psychological and creative therapies, neurosurgical interventions or genetics. Links with other disorders, such as autism spectrum disorder and Asperger syndrome, are being explored.

Family involvement in treatment

Eating disorders have an impact on family and carers as well as on the person with the illness. Eating disorders can cause enormous anxiety and distress for family members and carers, who worry about the health of their loved one and often feel frustrated, not knowing what to do to support them. They might feel alone, sometimes ashamed or as though they are to blame, and struggle to access support and treatment, as well as finding it hard to understand the illness.

Family and carers need support so that they can support the recovery journey and feel supported themselves. Naming the illness and using imagery can help this process. One young woman and her family used the idea of a menacing Jack-in-the-Box to represent her anorexia.

Body dysmorphic disorder

Christiana's story

Christiana, a 25-year-old hairdresser, has longstanding concerns about her nose. She dated this back to when she was at primary school and was teased about her 'big nose'. The concerns became overwhelming for her; she thought about it '24/7' and she started to miss school and social events because she worried that she was 'hideous'. She wore sunglasses to try to cover up the size of her nose, and pressured her parents into paying for cosmetic surgery when she turned 16. Initially, she was 'over the moon' about the results of the procedure, but soon started to think the surgeon had not taken enough off, and that it was now crooked. She had three more operations on her nose, but has never been happy with the outcome and now thinks her nose is too small. She is deeply distressed about this and is seeking legal redress from the surgeon. She repeatedly checks her reflection in the mirror, avoids socialising and does not work. She compares her nose to the noses of others and with images in magazines and on TV. Her mood is low and she is often tearful and has suicidal thoughts. She doesn't think life is worthwhile if she 'looks so awful'.

Over a series of appointments, she began to embrace the psychological aspects of her condition. Through treatment with cognitive–behavioural therapy and a selective serotonin reuptake inhibitor, she has returned to reasonable functioning.

Western cultures place a high value on physical appearance, and worries about body size and shape are very common, particularly for adolescent girls and young women. A recent Australian survey of nearly 50 000 people aged 11–24 years found that for a third of them, body image was one of their top three personal concerns. For 41% of young women, body image was their top concern, compared with 17% of young men (Mission Australia, 2016).

In body dysmorphic disorder, a woman is overly concerned about an aspect (or aspects) of her looks, apart from weight and shape. The physical 'flaws' are only slightly, or not at all, noticeable to others. The preoccupation might cause the woman considerable distress and affect her ability to function socially and get on with her life. She might engage in repetitive behaviours, such as spending a long time on her personal grooming, frequently checking her reflection in the mirror, or constantly comparing her appearance with that of others. Women with body dysmorphic disorder commonly seek reassurance from others about their appearance, but it never really helps them as they truly believe they are ugly.

There is less information in the public domain about body dysmorphic disorder than anorexia or bulimia. Body dysmorphic disorder commonly coexists with anorexia nervosa in women, highlighting how women have a tendency to overvalue appearance and to have a distorted way of seeing themselves.

Body dysmorphic disorder typically develops in adolescence. The areas of bodily concern tend to differ between women and men. Although the skin and parts of the face are areas of preoccupation in both genders, women are most often preoccupied with their stomach, hips, legs and chest (Phillips *et al*, 2006). Women with body dysmorphic disorder are more likely to also have an eating disorder than are men.

Women with body dysmorphic disorder see themselves as having a physical problem or defect that they believe can be 'fixed' by a procedure such as cosmetic surgery or dermatological fillers. The evidence is that such procedures, although often fine for women without this disorder, do not help women with the disorder. Cosmetic work tends to lead to an increase in the symptoms of body dysmorphic disorder, repeat procedures, expense and great unhappiness.

Treatment

Body dysmorphic disorder can be effectively treated with a combination of medication (mostly SSRI-type antidepressants) and psychological treatment. The psychological treatment usually includes cognitive–behavioural therapy, which aims to address both problem behaviours (e.g. excessive grooming, mirror-checking) and the underlying negative thinking that reinforces the disorder. Getting help from a psychologist or psychiatrist with expertise in the disorder, and not pursuing cosmetic 'cures', is critical.

Tips for women who think they might have an eating disorder or body dysmorphic disorder

If you are worried about your own body weight, size, or flaws, there are many ways to get help. Contact your general practitioner (GP) or hospital, or one of these organisations.

- Beat (www.b-eat.co.uk), the UK's leading eating disorder charity. Youth helpline: 0808 801 0711. Adult helpline: 0808 801 0677.

- Body Dysmorphic Disorder Foundation (www.bddfoundation.com)
- Mind (www.mind.org.uk)

Tips for family and friends

- If you are concerned that a woman might have an eating disorder or body dysmorphic disorder, encourage her to contact her GP or hospital without delay, or to access telephone and online support.
- Accessing specialist support early will maximise the chances of recovery from an eating disorder. A specialist team of clinicians, ideally including psychiatrists, medical physicians, dietitians, psychological therapists, specialist nurses and family therapists, can work together throughout the woman and her carers' journey, supported by voluntary and community sector organisations and schools.
- For young women (up to 18 years), new local, community eating disorder services are available across England (from April 2017). These will be accessible by self-referral/family referral, as well as referral from all agencies working with young people.

References and further reading

Anderson LH (2011) *Wintergirls*. Marion Lloyd Books.

Beat (2015) *The Costs of Eating Disorders: Social, Health and Economic Impacts*. Beat.

Honigman R, Castle DJ (2007) *Living With Your Looks*. University of Western Australia Press.

Koran LM, Aboujaoude E, Large MD, *et al* (2008) The prevalence of body dysmorphic disorder in the United States adult population. *CNS Spectrums*, **13**, 316.

Mission Australia (2016) *Youth Survey Report 2016*. Mission Australia.

National Institute for Health and Care Excellence (2004) *Eating Disorders: Core Interventions in the Treatment and Management of Anorexia Nervosa, Bulimia Nervosa and Related Eating Disorders* (CG9). NICE.

NHS Choices (2015) *Eating Disorders*. NHS (http://www.nhs.uk/conditions/Eating-disorders/Pages/Introduction.aspx).

Phillips KA (2005) *The Broken Mirror: Understanding and Treating Body Dysmorphic Disorder*. Oxford University Press.

Phillips KA, Menard W, Fay C (2006) Gender similarities and differences in 200 individuals with body dysmorphic disorder. *Comprehensive Psychiatry*, **47**, 77–87.

Rosen M (2013) The anorexic brain: neuroimaging improves understanding of eating disorder. *Science News,* **184**, 20–24.

Royal College of Psychiatrists (2012) *Junior MARSIPAN: Management of Really Sick Patients Under 18 with Anorexia Nervosa* (CR168). Royal College of Psychiatrists.

Royal College of Psychiatrists (2014) *MARSIPAN: Management of Really Sick Patients with Anorexia Nervosa* (CR189). Royal College of Psychiatrists.

Schmidt U, Treasure J, Alexander J (2015) *Getting Better Bite by Bite: A Survival Kit for Sufferers of Bulimia Nervosa and Binge Eating Disorders.* Routledge.

Treasure J (2007) *Skills-Based Learning for Caring for a Loved One with an Eating Disorder: The New Maudsley Method.* Routledge.

Psychosexual disorders

Jennifer Davies-Oliveira and Leila Frodsham

Mia's story

Mia is 33 years old and for the past 10 years she has suffered pain at the entrance to her vagina when having sex. She was very frightened when she arrived at the psychosexual clinic, didn't want to take off her coat, and sat with her bag on her knee ready to leave any minute. She was annoyed that her general practitioner (GP) had asked her to see a 'head doctor' and felt she just needs to be 'sorted' so that her partner can have sex with her. When the doctor told Mia that she was a gynaecologist, Mia burst into tears and told the doctor that she had been seen by six gynaecologists and had five operations so far: three to look into her womb and two to widen the entrance to her vagina, as well as several injections into her vagina. She had been given instruments to help her dilate her vaginal entrance, which she hated using and which caused her a lot of pain, even though she had been told the gel was an anaesthetic (so it wouldn't hurt). She also felt humiliated having to use them.

The pain she felt was so severe that she couldn't have sex with her partner who, although he loved her, had said he was no longer sure that his future is with her. They had stopped trying to achieve penetration as it was 'hopeless', and they were more like 'brother and sister' than romantic partners. She was extremely angry about the failure of her treatments to date, but remained convinced of a physical problem, saying it felt like there was a 'wall that stops him from getting in'.

On the examination couch, she drew her knees up and the cover to her chin. The doctor told her that the examination could wait and that Mia was 'in control' of the situation. She relaxed and allowed a finger in. Then she asked, 'What's it like … in there?'

The doctor asked if she would like to touch her vaginal area to find out. At first, Mia recoiled from the suggestion, but eventually she tentatively touched herself and remarked that it felt warm and safe. She began to cry as she revealed that her mother had told her never to touch herself 'down there' because it was 'dirty', and had also told her that she would feel pain and bleed when she first had sex. Mia was encouraged to massage her perineum regularly with oil and, at the next visit, reported that she had let her partner's finger in. At her next visit after that, she arrived in a colourful top with flowing hair (not her previous style) and shyly told the doctor that she had had sex without pain.

Pelvic pain and painful sexual intercourse

Problems with pelvic pain or painful sexual intercourse are known as genito-pelvic pain or penetration disorders. To be diagnosed with one or more of these problems, a woman would be experiencing significant distress associated with the following symptoms, which have occurred continually or repeatedly over 6 months.

- Fear or anxiety about pain in anticipation of, during, or after penetration.
- Difficulty with vaginal penetration.
- Tightening or tensing of the pelvic floor muscles during attempted penetration.
- Marked pain around the vagina and vulva or pelvic pain during penetration or attempted penetration.

Sexual pain is far more common than you might think, accounting for about 30% of all symptoms in women attending a gynaecology clinic (Nimnuan *et al*, 2001). The effects can vary greatly and it can be very distressing, leading to significant problems either starting or staying in relationships. Affected women can develop very low self-esteem and feelings of hopelessness, and even become depressed.

Sex involves both the mind and the body. The management of sexual pain is a perfect example of how to combine approaches to the body and the mind (Skrine & Montford, 2001).

Treatment

Women with genito-pelvic pain or penetration disorders often find it hard to tell a doctor what is going on or express what the underlying difficulty is. Ideally, the doctor will search for the trigger to a certain problem that the woman might not even be consciously aware of (Cowan & Frodsham, 2015). Specialist psychosexual doctors know that a woman needs to feel that they have been able to tell their story and that they have been listened to and believed (Kennedy & Moore, 2012). The patient will need to talk about details that might be difficult to disclose, such as when the pain started and whether this has any associations for the woman. For example, a woman's sexual pain might have started when she found out her partner had been unfaithful, when a family member became unwell, or because she feels guilty because of something she cannot express about her sex life or sexuality. The woman might not be aware that these things are connected with the onset of pain.

Therefore, the doctor will probably ask about other physical or emotional symptoms as well as previous treatments and whether they helped. Some women might have had surgery such as a diagnostic laparoscopy, which involves using a laparoscope to look inside the abdomen and pelvis for a physical cause of the pain, or a Fenton's procedure, which involves widening or stretching the vaginal entrance. These procedures are generally performed as day surgery in hospital, under anaesthetic.

It is important for the doctor to understand the woman's knowledge of sex and sexual experience and her family's attitudes to sexual behaviours (Crowley *et al*, 2009). Religious or family culture can underlie sexual difficulties, including sexual pain. A psychosexual specialist will be trained to understand that a woman could have experienced sexual or related trauma in her past and that this is an important issue in treatment.

Women who have experienced sexual abuse or rape can find it immensely difficult to tell a doctor intimate details about their relationship, their current and previous sex life, how they felt in their relationships and how they were treated. As you might expect, relationship problems are common in women with sexual pain, and they might need to explore the relationship difficulties as well as the sexual pain.

Although it can be frightening, having an intimate examination is vital in getting treatment for sexual pain. It can give the doctor insight into how the woman feels about intimacy and her genitals (Cowan & Frodsham, 2015). Mia felt fear related to her vulva and vagina, and this fear was related to how her mother had talked about Mia's vulva when she was young. Without a careful examination, taking into account the woman's feelings, fears and fantasies, she might never have experienced her 'moment of truth' and would have continued to experience sexual pain.

Surgery and other physical treatments

Despite an extensive search for a physical cause for the pain, in a significant proportion of women no such cause is found. Unfortunately, some doctors will continue to search for a physical cause for the pain. The result is that some women undergo unnecessary additional tests and surgeries, and do not get the care and treatment they actually need (Cowan & Frodsham, 2015). When investigating the cause of chronic pelvic pain, doctors should not use diagnostic laparoscopy in the first instance; they should only use it as a second-line investigation if other approaches have not identified the cause of the pain (Kennedy & Moore, 2012).

A study has shown that clinical staff who had psychosexual training and offered a holistic, psychodynamic consultation undertook no diagnostic laparoscopies as the first-line investigation (Davies & Frodsham, 2013). General gynaecologists, on the other hand, undertook this procedure in over two-thirds of women with sexual pain; in over half of the women who had a laparoscopy, no abnormalities were found (Davies & Frodsham, 2013). Often, a junior member of the day surgery team oversees the discharge of women who have negative laparoscopies, and women do not have a chance to explore the implications of the result for them. Women with a negative finding are likely to seek a second opinion, with the same outcome.

Other ways to manage chronic pain include local anaesthetics (e.g. lidocaine gel), but there is no evidence to support their use (Foster *et al*, 2010). Neither is there any support for the use of 'vaginal trainers' (intended to gradually accustom women to penetration) or neuromodulators (Vincent *et al*, 2015).

Tips for women with sexual pain

- Be curious about the pain and when it started. What was happening when it first came about?
- Try examining your genitals to become familiar with your own anatomy and examining where the pain is.
- Allow enough time for arousal and lubrication before intercourse. Use lubricants if needed (available off the shelf in supermarkets and pharmacies), as this can help with external sexual pain.
- Communicating with your partner can make them aware of your difficulties and help to lessen the pressure.
- Try to find a psychosexual doctor if you feel your pain needs further exploration. Take as much time as you need to talk to them about these difficult topics, which might be very upsetting to you.
- If you would prefer to speak to a woman, ask for a female physician (although this might not be possible).

Conclusions

A psychosexual element to sexual pain is very common. Psychosexual medicine brings psychological thinking to sexual disorders and provides a brief therapy exposing any unconscious thoughts, feelings and fantasies which can underpin a physical symptom (Skrine & Montford, 2001). This approach gives a holistic picture of the woman's sexual problem and helps tailor potential management options for her.

References and further reading

Cowan F, Frodsham L (2015) Management of common disorders in psychosexual medicine. *Obstetrician and Gynaecologist*, **17**, 47–53.

Crowley T, Goldmeier D, Hiller J (2009) Diagnosing and managing vaginismus. *BMJ*, **339**, 225–229.

Davies JC, Frodsham LCG (2013) Sex: what a pain! The investigation and management of sexual pain disorders in a district genecology department [abstract]. *BJOG*, **120** (Suppl 1), s490–s491.

Foster DC, Kotok MB, Huang LS, *et al* (2010) Oral desipramine and topical lidocaine for vulvodynia: a randomized controlled trial. *Obstetrics and Gynecology*, **116**, 583–593.

Kennedy SH, Moore SJ (2012) *The Initial Management of Chronic Pelvic Pain*. RCOG Press.

Nimnuan C, Hotopf M, Wessely S (2001) Medically unexplained symptoms: an epidemiological study in seven specialties. *Journal of Psychosomatic Research*, **51**, 361–367.

Skrine R, Montford H (2001) *Psychosexual Medicine: An Introduction* (2nd edn). Arnold.

Vincent KF, Curran N, Elneil S, *et al* (2015) *Therapies Targeting the Nervous System for Chronic Pelvic Pain Relief*. RCOG Press.

Personality disorders: risks and recovery

Gwen Adshead

Coralina's story

Coralina is a 27-year-old woman who went to her local mental health service after self-harming (cutting and overdosing). She said she heard a voice telling her to harm herself and others. She contacted Social Services because she was concerned that she might harm her 4-year-old daughter, but was very distressed when Social Services took her daughter into foster care.

Although Coralina had a long history of contact with mental health services, she had never been an in-patient, and she had always tried her best with the therapies and medications offered to her. She has looked up her symptoms on the internet and thinks she has borderline personality disorder; she wants help urgently and Social Services want an opinion about any risk to the child.

The psychiatrist asked detailed questions about Coralina's experience of herself, her life and her relationships with others. She asked about Coralina's experience of being cared for as a child, especially her experience of being looked after when ill, hurt or distressed. The psychiatrist assessed both Coralina's social functioning generally and her capacity to make and maintain relationships with partners, parents and siblings.

By doing this, the psychiatrist was looking at Coralina's strengths as well as vulnerabilities, trying to make an assessment of how severe the problems are, and the extent to which Coralina uses unhelpful, destructive coping strategies. She agreed with Coralina that the most likely diagnosis was a mild–moderate degree of borderline personality disorder. The good news was there are now a variety of evidence-based therapies that will help; the bad news was that Coralina's local NHS trust did not provide all of them and there was a long waiting list.

The psychiatrist agreed to support Coralina with regular psychiatric management while she waited for therapy. She also liaised with Social Services so that the work with Social Services and the psychiatric work with Coralina went hand in hand.

The initial period was stormy, but gradually Coralina began to trust her psychiatrist. She agreed to share care with the local authority. Her daughter was placed with family members who made it possible for Coralina to see her regularly and therefore maintain a good relationship with her. Eventually, Coralina got access to a specialist therapy group for mothers with borderline personality disorder, where she is making good progress.

What does your personality do?

Our personalities are a complex mixture of feelings, beliefs, values, thoughts and tendencies to action. These develop in childhood and continue to develop over time, although personalities change less as we get older.

Our personalities are made up of flexible elements that change in response to situations we find ourselves in and fixed elements that do not change much. The flexible elements help us deal with stress, pain and uncertainty in our lives, whereas the fixed elements allow others in our social or family group to recognise us.

Our personalities partly determine how we:

- manage the degree to which we get agitated and upset when we meet challenges and stress
- manage negative emotions and distress – especially how we experience those feelings in our bodies
- maintain an integrated sense of self over time, so that we are able to think about our own mind and the minds of others
- regulate relationships with the people on whom we depend (e.g. healthcare professionals, partners) or who depend on us (e.g. parents, children).

What is personality disorder?

Personality disorder is a term used to describe problems with personality functioning. Women with a personality disorder:

- struggle to manage negative feelings (e.g. distress, anger, sadness, anxiety); they may use drugs or alcohol to help them manage their feelings
- quickly become agitated if they feel stressed or threatened
- experience a lot of bodily discomfort (pain or sickness) and sometimes use their bodies to express distress (e.g. cutting, overdosing)
- find it hard to think about their own minds or the minds of others
- struggle to maintain close relationships with others, sometimes avoiding relationships altogether, or making very intense initial attachments to people, which then become negative.

Personality disorders are medical diagnoses. There are many listed in classification systems like the ICD-10 (1993) or the DSM-5 (2013). Overall, personality disorders are equally common in women and men, but borderline personality disorder might occur slightly more often in women and antisocial personality disorder more often in men (the evidence is mixed). The most common types of personality disorder are:

- borderline (or emotionally unstable) personality disorder
- antisocial personality disorder
- narcissistic personality disorder.

General practitioners (GPs) often refer women with these problems to mental health services because their personality dysfunction causes them problems with other people. But there are other personality disorders, which cause women to avoid social contact when they are distressed or cause them to retreat into a fantasy life. These women have as much distress as the others, but they are less visible.

What causes personality disorders?

The answer is complex and not completely known. Genes affect the development of our personalities, so genes are likely to have an influence on personality disorders too. However, we also know that early childhood trauma (especially physical abuse, neglect or emotional abuse) makes it more likely that a woman will develop a personality disorder. It is even possible for someone to develop a personality disorder after she has been through a major traumatic event in adulthood. We also know that mild degrees of personality disorder (which generally don't cause too much trouble) can become worse if women develop other mental illnesses, like depression or a psychotic disorder.

Why are we worried about women having personality disorders?

Living with a personality disorder is hard and distressing. It is also risky: women with a personality disorder have worse physical health as well as worse mental health, they frequently have problems with alcohol and drugs, and they are at increased risk of self-harm and suicide.

A small proportion of women with personality disorder pose a risk to others. This is mainly true for women with antisocial personality disorder, which is why many women with this kind of personality disorder are in prison. There is also a real problem for mothers with a personality disorder, because their distress has negative effects on their children. This does not mean that women with a personality disorder cannot have children, but they will need a lot of active help to manage the strong emotions that go with being a parent.

What can we do about it?

The good news is that treatments are available and they work well for people with mild to moderate degrees of personality disorder. Most treatment is offered on an out-patient basis. Women who can complete an appropriate treatment programme (which typically lasts about 18 months) can reduce self-harm and gain a sense of control over their feelings. Although they might relapse, many women with personality disorder make a good recovery and experience remission from most of their symptoms.

Sometimes women who cannot stop themselves self-harming will need admission to hospital. The evidence is that shorter stays are better. However, it is not uncommon for women who are self-harming badly to be admitted to specialist residential units for personality disorder, where they may stay for several months.

Treatment

There are two main therapies:

- dialectical behaviour therapy (DBT)
- mentalisation-based therapy (MBT).

There are other therapies available, such as schema-focused therapy and cognitive analytic therapy, but they aren't supported by such a high-quality evidence base.

The most effective therapies have a group component to them. Be wary of any therapist who claims that only individual work will help. Medication can have a useful role, especially at the beginning of therapy – this will usually be a mood stabiliser, antidepressant, or a low dose of an antipsychotic medication.

These treatments aim to make managing negative emotions and thoughts easier, and to improve the ability to see different perspectives in situations and with other people. Most of the treatment interventions will include some exploration of how childhood experiences might have influenced personality development. However, there is no evidence that therapies that focus exclusively on memories of past trauma are helpful, and they might make things worse.

The women who have the best outcomes are those who can stick with the treatment programmes. This is not always easy, and it is common for women attending personality disorder programmes to fall out with therapists, get angry or hopeless, and feel like giving up. It is very important to stick with the therapy even when it is difficult, because the potential benefits are huge. This is especially true for women who also have other problems, like eating disorders or substance misuse.

Tips for living with a personality disorder

- If you have experienced physical or emotional abuse and neglect in childhood, you might be at increased risk of developing a personality disorder.
- Living with a personality disorder is tough, but persistence is key.

- Look for and take advantage of self-help techniques (and professional therapies) to help you reduce self-harming behaviours.
- Good therapy won't take away your distress, but it should help empower you to manage it better.
- Short-term crisis admissions have been shown to have better outcomes than long-term in-patient stays.

Useful resource

Personality Disorders Awareness Network
www.pdan.org
Dedicated to increasing public awareness of personality disorders, helping families and preventing the development of personality disorders in children.

References and further rreading

American Psychiatric Association (2013) *Diagnostic and Statistical Manual of Mental Disorders, Fifth Edition*. APA.

Sarkar J, Adshead G (2006) Personality disorders as disorganisation of attachment and affect regulation. *BJPsych Advances*, **12**, 297–305.

Sarkar J, Adshead G (2012) *Clinical Topics in Personality Disorder*. RCPsych Publications.

World Health Organization (1993) *The ICD-10 Classification of Mental and Behavioural Disorders: Diagnostic Criteria for Research*. WHO.

Self-harm

Alys Cole-King and Sue Sibbald[†]

Self-harm is far more common than women realise, but it isn't talked about. Secrecy is the big enemy. We hope that this chapter will help women who use self-harm to understand more about their problems, to reduce or stop their self-harm and start their path to recovery, by 'talking not harming' and allowing themselves to feel supported by others.

What is self-harm?

Self-harm is when someone knowingly harms or injures themselves (Box 26.1). Some self-harm can cause immediate damage, other behaviours may be harmful in the longer term. Some people prefer the term self-injury. Other terms include deliberate self-harm or self-mutilation, but we urge people to stop using these terms – they are unhelpful, negative and contribute to stigma and judgemental attitudes. Words can make the pain worse and may delay the start of the healing and recovery process. Negative language can also discourage women from telling someone about their self-harm.

How common is self-harm?

Self-harm is an important health issue. It is more common in the UK than the rest of Europe. In the UK, approximately 6.5–8% of adolescents self-harm. This number drops to 4% in the adult population. Every year there are over 220000 attendances at hospital due to self-harm. The highest rates

---

[†]With a contribution from Andrea Woodside.

> **Box 26.1. Categories of self-harm**
>
> - *Direct self-harm*: an intentional act which causes immediate injury or harm to the body. No value judgement is made as to the motivation or degree of suicidal intent. This means it includes suicide attempts as well as acts where no suicidal intent is involved.
> - *Non-suicidal self-injury*: a term used to describe self-injury which emphasises the wish to deal with emotional pain rather than as a means for suicide, thus making it clear and distinct from other direct and indirect self-harming behaviours.
> - *Indirect self-harm*: covers a range of socially acceptable and unacceptable behaviours. These include smoking, drinking, drug-taking, eating disorders, and antisocial, risky, destructive and dangerous behaviours. As with direct self-harm, such behaviours are coping mechanisms to help deal with emotional distress; the frequency and danger increase as the distress worsens. These behaviours can be an indication that a person is in distress and could be at risk of more direct self-harm.

of self-harm are among young Black and South Asian women (Cooper *et al*, 2010).

Shame, embarrassment and fear of discovery mean that women often keep self-harm a secret unless they need medical treatment. Some may not tell anyone they self-harm simply because no one has ever asked them. As a result, we do not know the exact number of women who self-harm.

Women and self-harm

Self-harm is more common in women. Around 17% of girls and women will self-harm at some point in their lives, compared with 5% of men (Geulayov *et al*, 2016). There has been a rise in the number of women who attend hospital following self-harm associated with alcohol and drug misuse, possibly because drinking patterns in women are changing.

Why women self-harm

Self-harm is a sign of emotional distress, an indication that something is wrong rather than a symptom of a specific mental health issue or a mental 'disorder' itself. It is a way of trying to cope with difficult or intolerable emotions and situations. Unlike most book chapters or articles about self-harm, we are not listing all the various types of self-harm. We think that professionals need to focus on the person in distress, their reasons for self-harm and how they can be best supported on their way to recovery. However, we need to highlight that some people who self-harm need urgent medical attention, especially if the self-harm includes an overdose. This will usually involve a trip to the nearest emergency department. Advice on who to contact if you are unsure what to do can be found in Box 26.3 at the end of this chapter.

The underlying reasons for self-harm are different for each woman (some are listed in Box 26.2). Women who self-harm experience negative emotions, such as anxiety, depression

---

Box 26.2. Reasons for self-harm

- Expression of personal distress – often due to unbearably intense emotional distress (a 'bright red scream')
- Concealment of distress (a 'private pain')
- Desperation (inability to cope with overwhelming emotional or physical pain any longer)
- To 'stay alive' as it is the only thing that gives a relief from distressing thoughts and feelings of suicide
- Trauma or abuse (often relating to childhood experiences)
- Poor self-esteem, self-hatred, guilt, belief that punishment is needed
- Isolation, lack of a sense of belonging
- To 'feel real', i.e. validation of existence acquired through sight of blood or feeling pain
- To provide a sense of control or increased control if the individual feels they have no control in their life
- Escalation of less concerning injuries or behaviours
- To act out the care that the individual would like to be shown (e.g. to enable the woman to self-care in a way that she would not normally do so, for instance dressing the wounds)
- Being in a minority group
- To make the body less attractive (can be related to abusive experiences)

Source: Connecting with People. Reprinted with permission
(www.connectingwithpeople.org)

and impulsivity, more frequently than those who do not self-harm. They might also have difficulties with expressing their emotions, solving their problems and self-esteem. Some women who self-harm report that their feelings were 'invalidated' in childhood – that is, certain feelings were not allowed, categorised as wrong or bad, or resulted in punishment. For some people, trauma is at the root of self-harm and there is a growing body of research showing that trauma-informed care is a vital part of recovery.

For some women, self-harm is a coping mechanism to help them resist acting on long-term suicidal thoughts. In rare cases, women who self-harm do go on to end their lives, making it important that we take self-harm seriously. For a small minority, self-harm could be related to a serious mental illness.

Stopping using self-harm as a coping strategy

Many women self-harm only once during a particularly stressful situation. Women with good emotional and social support, who know they have people who care about them, are less likely to consider self-harm or ending their lives. If women have self-harmed for some time, they may need more support, including help from a specialist voluntary organisation or a professional. If the person who self-harms is under 18, and especially if they are under 16, it is important they find support from an adult they trust.

Building emotional well-being and resilience

Most of us manage our physical health better than our emotional health, leaving problems or ongoing concerns to cause potential harm. Resilience refers to a person's ability to cope with everyday difficulties and not feel too badly affected by them. Emotional resilience is the ability to cope with stressful situations and adapt to the ups and downs of life. Emotional resilience is not about 'mental toughness' but about having enough emotional, social and internal strategies to deal with difficult situations. It is not about asking women to 'grin and bear it' or to handle impossible situations.

Ways to build resilience:

- try to notice when you start to get stressed or upset – and take action, the earlier the better

- write a 'worry list' of what is bothering you – break it down into small, manageable parts and tackle each one at a time
- the key is to cope with things one day at a time.

Everyone can make a personal plan to increase well-being and ability to cope. Encourage a woman who uses self-harm to do this. Taking time to do things for ourselves can feel selfish, but it's important to look after ourselves to help our emotional well-being. Self-care is not selfish, far from it – self-care is vital.

Visit the U Can Cope and Staying Safe webpages (see the 'Useful resources' section at the end of the chapter) for more information.

Treatment strategies

Women who have used self-harm need treatment and the same level of compassion, kindness, care, respect and privacy as any other patient. Self-harm is a behaviour, not an illness. Treatment depends on identifying the underlying cause of the distress and seeing the woman, not just the self-harm. Every contact with a woman who uses self-harm is a chance to address the unbearable emotional distress that she is feeling. Treatment goals should be to support her to develop less harmful ways of coping with distress.

Some women try to reduce their self-harm by removing the means for self-harm. This is an individual decision and women need person-centred support, including a safety plan (Box 26.3, pp. 175–176). It is never too late to take action to help a situation that seems hopeless. Some women manage fairly easily to stop feeling as if they need to self-harm, but others do not. If this is the case, try to support them to look at harm reduction in the meantime until they feel ready to try to stop.

Hear from women who use self-harm

1.

Hello Distress,

I can't say I've missed you, as familiar as you are, but there you were at the door last night, your insistent knock telling me that you'd let yourself in if I didn't. The door opened, filling the hallway with your dark shadow, although your features were recognisable because they never change. Frozen to my spot, I fell through the wounds you've inflicted over the years.

'It's been a long time', you said, turning your head to see if I was alone. You moved towards me just slowly enough to draw out the torture. Night fell as the street lights flickered out, my fear melting me.

You first knocked at the door when I was 7 years old. A child hoping that something, anything, would end an interminable pain. An innocent mind which should never have known of these things, I thought I'd found a friend to lead me confidently out of the hell. But you were not a friend. Instead, shrill voices told me that they were inconvenienced by a childish recklessness, blaming me for something they could not understand.

I have lived with you peering over my shoulder for many years, your need to win at times drowning everything else out. But there is always one molecule in my body, hidden at times even from me, that keeps me here. You are not big enough to win against my will to survive, to hold hope, to live.

Dear Hope,

Despite the sometimes unrelenting distress, you come to me in many forms, feeling your way through the darkness to reach me. I marvel now at the way in which you have always been here, although at times I could only see your outline, hazy but formed. You're always here, waiting patiently to unlock the door, like a locksmith whose key remains new and perfect. You have kept me here long after my 7th birthday. You were my godmother throughout my childhood, knowing that something was trying to claim me, and whilst the language of distress was not her mother tongue, she wrested me back with compassionate words, looks and hugs, learning a language that must have been at times overwhelming to her.

You were a teacher at my school who spent time telling me I was good at so many things, that I had a future full of wonder to come. You were – and continue to be – a moment standing in a summer's field, leaving me marvelling at the wonder of being connected to its calming warmth. You are the person sitting across from me on a train journey, hurtling at speed towards unfamiliar places, a fellow being who perhaps has felt the same at times but is testament to how hope never lies. You are the psychiatrist who shows me a way to tenderly hold my heart, reminding me that it defends against arrows which cannot puncture, despite their single-minded trajectory.

Your track record of extending inexhaustible hope is 100%. My track record of seeing through the darkness until your form is crystalline is 100%. We share a common aim, swifter than arrows can ever fly. You are all those who walk with me shoulder to shoulder, shining their brilliant beams ahead of me despite the odds. Together, we bring in the light.

Although, from time to time, distress attempts to embezzle what tells me to stay, you, hope, win every time, reminding me that the pain will dissipate like smoke from a fire. The pain has not won. I am alive. I am alive.

Andrea Woodside

2.

I began to self-harm at an early age. I'd had a difficult childhood and as I'm a woman in her fifties now I didn't realise what I was doing was self-harm. Nobody talked about mental health in my days and self-harm was a taboo subject.

In my teens, my self-harm became worse but I lived with a nurse who would look after me. I avoided hospitals and anything to do with mental health as I didn't see anything wrong with what I was doing and I had a fear of psychiatrists as my mother had schizophrenia and was locked up often. I feared the same happening to me.

I took drugs as a form of self-harm at this time, also to blot out having to feel anything. I never reflected until recently about the function of my self-harm back then but I think now that I couldn't face my past and the hurt I kept reliving in my life in the here and now. I was triggered but wasn't aware what was happening. I hid my self-harm from everyone.

Later in my 40s I became quite ill and got referred to secondary mental health. My self-harm was much worse, I was very dissociative and suffered with extreme anxiety and depression. I would self-harm both as a form of self-harm and a couple of times with intent to end my life.

However, I became determined to try to help myself and taught myself a therapy called DBT [dialectical behaviour therapy]. Within the skills that you learn are ways to help if you feel like self-harming like distracting, being mindful of emotions as they rise, so you can manage them or sit with them.

I personally use such things as walking, the gym, gardening, playing Angry Birds, sitting with my children and being busy with work. If I'm feeling strong urges to self-harm, I go and do some really tough physical exercise or try some paced breathing.

I very rarely self-harm now. It has to be something huge in my life to trigger me and I do so in a way that's not dangerous. I prefer my life now too as I did feel terrible personal shame around my self-harm and having to hide scars sometimes feels embarrassing for me.

One day I am hopeful I will stop altogether but for now I'm in acceptance I'm on the right path. I will get there.

Sue Sibbald

Tips for women who are distressed and feel a need to self-harm

You can help yourself in lots of ways. You can start by making a 'safety plan' (Box 26.3) for yourself as soon as possible. It includes what you can do for yourself and to whom you can speak if you need support. It will be useful because you will have chosen the kind of support that you feel comfortable with.

Tips for family and friends

Changes in behaviour, especially isolation from family and friends and not joining in with usual activities, might be a sign of a problem. A change to wearing covered-up clothing (that can hide marks and scars) might be a sign that a woman is self-harming.

The good news is that, with support, young women who self-harm can develop better ways of coping and, in the young, it tends to resolve as they grow up. Talking instead of harming is vital on the road to recovery. The most important thing is to let her know you care.

Ways to build trust

- Provide a safe environment that is free from disruption.
- Remain calm and caring, and avoid panic and overreaction.
- Use open body language, appropriate eye contact and active listening, and tell her you know how difficult things must be right now.
- Avoid statements that they could perceive as minimising their distress such as 'Surely it's not that bad' or 'Come on now... you need to get over this'.
- Take a no-blame approach (i.e. accept her, even if you disagree with her behaviour).
- Know that this represents a way of dealing with emotional pain.
- Try not to show shock or revulsion at what she has done.
- Do not use threats in an attempt to stop the behaviour.
- Know that you are not responsible for her self-harm and look after yourself too – it can be upsetting when someone you care about uses self-harm to cope with distress.

Box 26.3   Making a safety plan

Reasons for living and/or ideas for getting through tough times

- Reminders of positive aspects of your life: photos of people, pets or places you care about.
- Music that boosts your mood and makes you feel good.

Making your situation safer

- Remove things you could use to harm yourself.
- If stopping self-harm is not an option yet, can you make the self-harm safer?
- Can you identify and avoid things that you know make you feel worse? These are called *distress triggers*.

Things to lift or calm your mood

- A calming activity is anything you find relaxing.
- Meditation, yoga or looking at a photo of a great view or someone you care about.
- Write your feelings down in a diary or a letter – sometimes it is easier to write things down than tell someone how you are feeling.
- Calming thoughts such as about a special place or happy memory.

Distractions – activities to take your mind away from your distressing feelings

- Distracting activities (e.g. listening to music, exercise, cooking, art).
- Distract your thoughts by keeping your mind busy (e.g. crosswords or sudoku).

Sources of support can include anyone you trust

- Day-to-day support (not necessarily for discussing self-harm)
  - agree to talk to someone you trust, including friends, family or people in your community.
- Support if you are distressed or thinking about self-harm
  - specialist support such as from helplines or mental health professionals.
- Specific suicide and self-harm prevention 24-hour helplines or websites
  - local healthcare support, emergency NHS contact details for out-of-hours support.
- If you can, write down all contact details so that you have them when you need them – include home/work/mobile numbers:
  - family
  - friends – include their name and phone number
  - anyone close to where you live

Cont.

- a list of specialist suicide prevention helplines, social media sites and websites
- your own family doctor and a number to reach the doctor's surgery out of hours. Your mental healthcare professional or peer support workers from a mental health team or care coordinator if you have one.

- Social media
  - Social media can be a good way to find out how others have learned to cope with their urge to self-harm. Consider finding a local peer-support group or, if you are active on social media, join a chatroom or Facebook group, or make contact with others via Twitter. Not all chatrooms are moderated as closely as they might be, so if you find one triggering or upsetting then perhaps avoid that one in the future. Sue Sibbald, one of the authors of this chapter, has created a weekly Tweetchat on Twitter called #BPDChat. People from around the UK (and beyond) gather online to offer valuable support to each other.

Source: Connecting with People. Reprinted with permission (www.connectingwithpeople.org)

Important points

- If you have already self-harmed it's still OK to make a safety plan – it's never too late.
- If you are a young person under 18, and especially if you are under 16, please find support from an adult you can talk to and trust – don't feel that you have to cope with all your problems alone.
- If you are already supported by a health professional, tell them how you are feeling and show them your safety plan, even if they haven't asked to see it.
- Be kind to yourself and always remember that however you feel, you are worthy of help and support.
- Remember that things can change. What you are going through right now is really tough but you can get through it. Please remember – never give up.

Useful resources

Mental Health Foundation
www.mentalhealth.org.uk/help-information/mental-health-a-z/S/self-harm

Staying safe if you're not sure life's worth living
www.connectingwithpeople.org/StayingSafe
Online support for anyone who is struggling. It offers hope, compassion and practical ideas to get through tough times.

Tips for self-care
www.connectingwithpeople.org/content/mhaw17

U Can Cope
www.connectingwithpeople.org/ucancope
U Can Cope is designed to help young people develop resilience and cope with current and future difficulties in their life, but it is just as helpful for adults.

References and further reading

Cole-King A, Green G, Wadman S, *et al* (2011) Therapeutic assessment of patients following self-harm. *InnovAiT*, **4**, 278–287.

Cooper J, Murphy E, Webb R, *et al* (2010) Ethnic differences in self-harm, rates, characteristics and service provision: three-city cohort study. *British Journal of Psychiatry*, **197**, 212–218.

Geulayov G, Kapur N, Turnbull P, *et al* (2016) Epidemiology and trends in non-fatal self-harm in three centres in England, 2000–2012: findings from the Multicentre Study of Self-harm in England. *BMJ Open*, **6**, e010538.

National Institute for Health and Care Excellence (2011) *Self-Harm: Longer-Term Management* (CG133). NICE.

Ness J, Hawton K, Bergen H, *et al* (2015) Alcohol use and misuse, self-harm and subsequent mortality: an epidemiological and longitudinal study from the multicentre study of self-harm in England. *Emergency Medical Journal*, **32**, 793–799.

Royal College of Psychiatrists (2010) *Self-Harm, Suicide and Risk: Helping People who Self-Harm* (CR158). Royal College of Psychiatrists.

Women and addiction

Sally Marlow

Luisa's story

Luisa is in her mid-40s and the mother of two children, Megan (17) and Dan (14). For as long as she can remember she's been drinking wine most evenings with dinner, but at some point she began to drink earlier, when preparing supper, and recently she has had her first drink at around 4 pm. She now drinks every day. She typically has a bottle of wine a night, but these days even that doesn't seem to have an effect, so she will open a second bottle. She thinks she probably drinks too much, and has tried to cut down several times, but without success.

Luisa was a trainee accountant who liked to party when she met her husband Mark in a nightclub. At 25, she became unexpectedly pregnant with Megan and, as soon as she realised, cut down on her drinking to one or two glasses of wine a week. After Megan was born, she and Mark married, and Dan followed soon after.

Mark was a dominant husband and made it clear that he wanted Luisa to be a full-time mother. He would get home from work after Luisa had put the children to bed, then they would eat together, usually with wine. Four years ago, Mark left, after what Luisa thinks was an unhappy marriage. Luisa has since found a part-time job doing the accounts for a local group of dentists.

Recently, she's started to get pains in her stomach, feels shaky in the afternoons and has gone from looking forward to the first drink of the day to wanting it; she now feels she needs it. Getting up in the mornings is increasingly difficult and she has been late for work several times. Megan, meanwhile, is going through what Luisa calls a 'difficult phase' – she's out every night, sometimes not coming home. Luisa knows Megan is drinking and smoking, and suspects it may be cannabis as well as tobacco. At weekends she and her friends 'pre-load' on cheap spirits in Megan's bedroom before they go out clubbing. Luisa doesn't mind this – she'd rather they were doing it under her roof than somewhere else and she remembers the heady days of her late teens, when she was doing much the same herself.

Dan seems okay, but Luisa doesn't really know – he doesn't talk to her much, which makes her vaguely uneasy. In fact, she doesn't feel she has an emotional connection with either of her children, but by the end of the day she doesn't have the energy to make much effort. She wonders if she might be depressed.

Alcohol is not the only drug that causes problems for women, but it is by far the most common. Luisa's story illustrates the complicated relationship between addiction and life events, physical health, mental health and gender roles in women, as well as the impact it can have on their children.

When is a woman 'addicted'?

The word 'addiction' has been adopted into everyday language, with people talking about being addicted to a TV series, or being a 'chocoholic'. However, this minimises what addiction really is: a condition that is sufficiently serious and distressing as to be treated as a psychiatric disorder by the medical community and that can bring severe mental and physical health problems, and even death. It is possible to be addicted not only to substances like alcohol and drugs, but also to behaviours such as gambling and possibly even eating. To complicate matters further, there are degrees of addiction severity.

Alcohol addiction ranges from regular (but sporadic) excessive, risky drinking (often referred to as binge drinking or heavy episodic drinking), through a pattern of drinking that is causing harm to the drinker and/or those around them, to what clinicians refer to as dependence (World Health Organization, 1993). Signs that a woman is dependent on a substance can be physical, such as needing more and more of the substance to achieve the same effect, or having severe withdrawal symptoms such as shaking, headaches, stomach pains and nausea. These can be seen in the case of Luisa, who also shows some of the psychological signs of addiction, including cravings, lack of control, an inability to give up or cut down, not being able to fulfil what's expected of you (in her case both at work and at home) and persisting despite knowing it is doing you harm.

Which women are most at risk of addiction?

Addiction is genetic to some extent, with around 100 genes probably playing a part. Although a woman might be genetically vulnerable to addiction problems, this doesn't mean that she is destined to develop them, as genes are not the whole story. There are also environmental factors that can contribute; these include a crisis or stressful life event, which can act as a trigger. In Luisa's case, a clear link can be seen between Mark leaving and her drinking increasing, almost as though she was using the alcohol to self-medicate the pain (Khantzian, 1997). Marriage seems to protect women from running into problems with drink and drugs, but separation or divorce seems to do the opposite.

The story of Luisa's alcohol use and her daughter Megan's excessive drinking also demonstrates a key point about addiction: it tends to run in families (Agrawal & Lynskey, 2008). This is because of both genetic and environmental factors that are present in families. Children might inherit genes that make them vulnerable, but also learn that the excessive drink and drug use they see in their parents is normal. They might also have psychological and behavioural problems resulting from poor parenting.

This complicated mix contributes to the fact that the children of parents with addiction problems are more likely to drink and use drugs excessively themselves. Mothers are the primary caregivers in many families and, as Luisa's story demonstrates, a woman's excessive use of alcohol might have consequences not only for her, but also for her children. Luisa seems blunted to the needs of Megan and Dan: this lack of emotional availability can be difficult to spot, but is common among mothers with addiction problems.

Addiction, depression and abuse

Depression is often found in women with addiction problems, much more so than in men (Dawson *et al*, 2010). However, it is sometimes difficult to work out whether the depression leads to addiction problems, or vice versa. When domestic abuse is also part of a depressed woman's life, the combination of the abuse, depression and addiction is referred to by some as the 'toxic trio'. Together, these create a vicious circle – the greater the abuse, the greater the depression and the greater the addiction problems (Heise, 2011). Domestic abuse does not have to be physical – emotional abuse can often be damaging for women, and Luisa's case hints at this when Mark's controlling nature is described.

Alcohol-related damage and the 'telescope effect'

As a group, women have fewer problems with addiction than men: they drink less and fewer women than men take illicit drugs. However, women are sometimes more likely than men to develop addiction problems with prescription painkillers and tranquilisers.

Addiction problems, and the physical and psychological damage that accompany them, can develop over a woman's lifespan. Luisa partied hard at weekends when she was younger, and now in middle age has developed a daily pattern of heavy drinking. Contrary to stories in the media, the women who may be most at risk of alcohol-related harm are in their 40s, not young women out on the town on a Friday night. Those younger women do, however, run risks at the time of excessive drinking, including accidents and alcohol poisoning.

Most women cut back on drinking (and drug-taking) in their mid-to-late 20s, but for those who do not, like Luisa, as addiction starts to take hold, their brains and bodies adapt to cope with alcohol or other drugs and the damage can be longer lasting – in some cases, permanent. That damage can include liver disease and increased risks of cancer, dementia, reproductive problems and stroke, along with mental health problems. A cruel trick of biology means that women's bodies develop these harms earlier and more severely in their lives, and having consumed less of a substance than men. This is sometimes called the 'telescope effect' (Diehl *et al*, 2007).

Treating women with addiction problems

Treatment is often complicated by the high rates of depression and other problems in women with addiction. A further complication in women with children is that there may be effects on her family to take into account; for example, although residential rehabilitation might be the best treatment choice for a particular woman, it would require her to leave her family for 3–6 months, which is often difficult to achieve. Treatment programmes for women should therefore be holistic, taking into account the complex needs of each woman, and in extreme cases may also need to address social issues, such as housing and support back into the workplace.

A pregnant woman with addiction problems requires intensive support from specialist midwives, doctors and social workers, alongside addiction professionals, as there is often a danger that the substances she is using can damage the fetus.

Access to different treatments varies and, despite extensive lobbying over the years for women-only programmes, few exist. In addition, getting women into treatment for addiction is difficult as they face enormous stigma and women with children might fear that if they seek help, they will lose their children. However, once in treatment, women can respond well, and with the right support find a way out of their addiction and the problems that go with it.

References and further reading

Agrawal A, Lynskey MT (2008) Are there genetic influences on addiction: evidence from family, adoption and twin studies. *Addiction*, **103**, 1069–1081.

Dawson DA, Goldstein RB, Moss HB, *et al* (2010) Gender differences in the relationship of internalizing and externalizing psychopathology to alcohol dependence: likelihood, expression and course. *Drug and Alcohol Dependence*, **112**, 9–17.

Diehl A, Croissant B, Batra A, *et al* (2007) Alcoholism in women: is it different in onset and outcome compared to men? *European Archives of Psychiatry and Clinical Neuroscience*, **257**, 344–351.

Heise LL (2011) *What Works to Prevent Partner Violence: An Evidence Overview*. London School of Hygiene and Tropical Medicine.

Khantzian EJ (1997) The self-medication hypothesis of substance use disorders: a reconsideration and recent applications. *Harvard Review of Psychiatry*, **4**, 231–244.

World Health Organization (1993) *The ICD-10 Classification of Mental and Behavioural Disorders: Diagnostic Criteria for Research*. WHO.

Autism spectrum disorder

Helen Pearce

Autism spectrum disorder (ASD) is a neurodevelopmental disorder – a disorder of 'wiring'. This means people with ASD process information in a way that is different from the 'neuro-typical' population. Currently, internationally agreed criteria define ASD as a developmental disorder with difficulties in two key domains:

- difficulties in social communication and reciprocal social interactions
- difficulties in social imagination and restricted, repetitive and stereotyped behaviours and interests, along with sensory sensitivities.

ASD is a broad disorder within a broader-still group of disorders known as the pervasive developmental disorders. In recent years, professionals, affected families and the general public have become aware that there is a range of ASD disorders and that affected individuals can be at any point 'on a spectrum'. Our understanding of the nature of the difficulties that affected people have is always evolving. Classification and guidelines for clinical judgement continue to develop and change.

For some people, their difficulties related to autism are clear for others to see – they stand out. For others, their outward difficulties may be much more subtle, even if the impact is still enormous. The definition of ASD has broadened and, without doubt, this has led to some loss of clarity.

Women with ASD have historically been underdiagnosed, particularly those who manage to function well. Concern has been growing that girls and women with ASD might be overlooked within the new frameworks.

Different presentations in women

ASD often presents differently in women and men. This can result in delays in diagnosis of women, as their symptoms are not considered 'typical'. There is increasing evidence that the assessment tools used for diagnosis are inherently biased towards the signs and symptoms men tend to show. William Mandy and David Skuse have explored this in some detail. In 2015, they joined to present a webinar on the current understanding of gender differences in 'the female autism conundrum'.

Women with ASD might have developed better superficial social skills than men and this can mask the level of social deficit, unless a doctor digs deeper. Many high-functioning women and girls with ASD are never referred for assessment, and therefore never diagnosed, even though they are equally in need of treatment and support.

Girls and women who are more 'able' tend to learn how to blend in to a greater extent than boys and men, who can struggle in this area. In addition, they tend to demonstrate obsessional behaviours and interests that are more in keeping with social norms, so they are less likely to stand out as unusual or different from their peers.

However, many girls and women with ASD can feel socially ostracised and do not fit into a peer group well. They might be able to form initial relationships but struggle to develop them. They do not tend to fit into classic pictures of the difficulties that characterise ASD. Many girls and women with ADS have an ability to develop a single friendship or smaller groups of friends, and can be socially protected if they are accepted by a small social circle. Others, however, never achieve this, which can create isolation and distress.

Differential diagnosis

ASD can mask or mimic a wide range of other psychiatric problems. Many girls and women visit medical professionals with difficulties, but these might be misunderstood and labelled incorrectly as symptoms of other mental disorders. Although having ASD as an underlying difficulty doesn't mean a woman won't develop other mental disorders (indeed, anxiety and depression are more likely in those who struggle), it is not uncommon for more able women with ASD to be misdiagnosed with other difficulties. They might have difficulty with emotional regulation and anxiety, resulting in a misdiagnosis of personality difficulties or personality disorder.

Changes in assessments

Research suggests high-functioning women and girls with ASD have been underdiagnosed compared with men and boys. This can lead to difficulties in accessing sufficient assessment and subsequent appropriate support. When assessing girls and women, medical professionals need to understand how this group might present differently, and adapt and extend the assessments accordingly.

Women with ASD who inspire

Women and girls with ASD, like anyone else, need to understand themselves and who they are as individuals, so that they can develop to their full potential. They face the added question of whether ASD plays a part in their personalities.

Some women with ASD have become well known for the difficulties they have overcome and what they have achieved. There are too many to list, but the women mentioned below are a particular inspiration to other women with ASD, and indeed medical professionals, in the way they have educated others on their condition and become advocates for other women with ASD. Some have faced adversity and some continue to struggle, but all have shown great determination in seeking the lives they wish to follow.

Temple Grandin

Temple Grandin is a professor at Colorado State University, an expert in animal science and the humane handling of livestock. As a child, she was diagnosed with autism and deemed by doctors to be unable to achieve. Yet her success has been awe-inspiring, so much so that her story has been captured on film for others to learn from. Read more about Temple at her website (www.templegrandin.com).

Robyn Steward

Robyn Steward is an award winning specialist trainer, musician, artist, broadcaster and mentor. She has a form of autism called Asperger syndrome. I have had the pleasure of speaking at conferences alongside Robyn. Her journey has been traumatic at times, but she has overcome her difficulties to teach and educate others in the way that she has navigated life and learnt to use her extraordinary gifts to teach others to open their eyes and learn. Find out more about her story at her website (www.robynsteward.com).

Alis Rowe

Alis Rowe has Asperger syndrome. She is an entrepreneur and author. In 2013, she founded 'The Curly Hair Project', a social enterprise which supports women and girls with autism. Alis has struggled throughout her life in ways that have motivated her to help others understand and appreciate how it might be to cope with everyday situations and the obstacles in life that the 'neurotypical' population cannot easily imagine. She shares her experiences and 'conundrums' that arise from surviving everyday life as a woman with Asperger's on her website (https://thegirlwiththecurlyhair.co.uk).

Donna Williams

Donna Williams is a writer, artist, sculptor and singer songwriter. She has autism but was originally diagnosed with 'childhood psychosis'. She reminds us she is a person who has achieved and gained success rather than a person with ASD who has struggled. It is a lesson to read her words:

> '... if I'm going to have conditions I can't get rid of then I'd rather integrate their associated challenges into my daily life so I can get on with focusing on my personhood as a human being among the wide colourful diversity that is humankind.'

Learn more about Donna and her story at her website (www.donnawilliams.net).

Useful resources

National Autistic Society
www.autism.org.uk/about/what-is/gender.aspx
Information on gender and autism

The female autism conundrum, a webinar by W. Mandy & D. Skuse. Available at https://spectrumnews.org/features/webinars/webinar-the-female-autism-conundrum/ (accessed 23 May 2017).

Attention-deficit hyperactivity disorder

Gaelle Slater and Helen Crimlisk

Ruth's story

Ruth is a 32-year-old woman. She left school at 16, having got into trouble for not working hard enough, arguing and getting into fights with other girls. She had a stormy relationship with her mother, who said she was a difficult child, 'into everything and could have done better if she had tried'. She has lost several jobs in retail for getting angry with customers, but more recently has enjoyed working as a gardener in a small firm. She is disorganised at home, struggling to keep on top of things, and this resulted in her relationship ending. Her 7-year-old son was getting into trouble at school, has dyslexia and has recently been diagnosed with attention-deficit hyperactivity disorder (ADHD). Medication has helped him in his school work and his behaviour at school and at home. She asked her general practitioner (GP) for referral to an adult ADHD specialist, and was subsequently diagnosed with ADHD, which made a lot of sense to her. She tried medication but, although this helped, it also caused side-effects. She has read a lot about ADHD and manages her symptoms better as a result of developing better coping strategies, and by avoiding or planning for situations that might cause conflict.

ADHD stands for 'attention-deficit hyperactivity disorder'. You might also have heard of the terms 'hyperkinetic disorder' or 'attention-deficit disorder'. These all describe a similar condition, in which people have difficulties with concentration and focusing and can be overactive.

The symptoms of ADHD are similar in women and men, and it is diagnosed and treated in the same way for most people. There is some evidence that women are less likely to have hyperactivity symptoms and predominantly experience problems with concentration and attention. Women are diagnosed with

ADHD four times less often than men, although we do not know whether this reflects a real difference in prevalence or whether ADHD is simply recognised less often in women.

ADHD is a developmental disorder, which means it starts in childhood and often continues into adult life. It is not usually diagnosed before 6 years of age, as many children below this age are naturally very active and cannot focus on things for a long time. As they mature, children's brains develop the ability to concentrate for longer and focus on one thing at a time. Girls with ADHD do not develop this ability at the same rate and might struggle, particularly in the classroom environment, at home and socially. ADHD can continue into adult life and some women struggle with the symptoms throughout their lives.

What causes ADHD?

We don't know exactly what causes ADHD. We do know that it seems to run in families: a third of people with ADHD have at least one parent with similar symptoms. This suggests that ADHD is passed on through the genes we get from our parents; however, it's a complex picture and it's not just one gene that is responsible.

It's likely that some parts of the brain develop slightly differently in women with ADHD, and for this reason these women might have an imbalance in the chemicals that help us to concentrate (neurotransmitters). The treatments for ADHD change the balance of these chemicals and can reduce the severity of symptoms. ADHD is more likely to occur in women who have other conditions, such as intellectual disability, autism spectrum disorder, epilepsy and tics.

Although parents can feel guilty, as if they have somehow caused their child to develop ADHD, we know that children from any background can develop the disorder. It is not caused by poor parenting, although children with good parental support might manage their symptoms better; this is something the family can learn.

What does it feel like?

Women with ADHD can have a variety of symptoms that affect their behaviour. These include:

- having a short attention span and being easily distracted (inattention)
- being overactive and struggling to keep still (hyperactivity)
- doing things without thinking of the consequences (impulsivity).

Not everyone with ADHD has the same symptoms. Some people experience concentration difficulties but do not seem to be physically overactive; this is sometimes referred to as attention-deficit disorder and seems to be more common in women.

We all differ in our ability to concentrate and in how active we are. Some women might recognise some of the symptoms described but feel that they add something positive to their personality. We would not say that they had ADHD unless the symptoms happened most of the time, no matter what environment they were in, and they had a significant negative impact on their ability to live life normally.

Difficulties with concentration and being overactive can cause other problems for women with ADHD. They can have outbursts of anger, experience mood swings or become easily frustrated. Listening to instructions can be difficult and they can find it hard to wait their turn. They can be disorganised, easily forget things, move from one task to the next and struggle to finish things. Being impulsive can also lead to women doing risky or dangerous things without thinking about the consequences. They might get in trouble at home, at school or with the police as a result. Young people with ADHD can be labelled as 'naughty'. Some woman can feel stigmatised by the way that others see their behaviour, and this can affect their self-esteem and make it difficult to make friends.

It is difficult for any adult with ADHD to balance home and work life, but for mothers with ADHD, the added role of caring for and organising a family can make life very stressful. Forgetfulness, disorganisation and difficulty finishing tasks are common in ADHD, and trying to coordinate and support others can be especially hard. It can be even tougher if there are also children with ADHD in the home.

Signs you might have ADHD

- You get easily distracted and find it hard to take notice of details, particularly with things you find boring.

- It's hard to listen to other people – you find yourself interrupting, or saying things at the wrong time.
- It's hard to follow instructions.
- You are forgetful and tend to lose or misplace things.
- It's hard to organise yourself, and you start a lot of things without finishing them.
- It's hard to wait and you get bored easily – you fidget and can't sit still.
- You get easily irritated, impatient or frustrated and lose your temper quickly.
- You feel restless or edgy, have difficulty turning your thoughts off and find stress hard to handle.
- You tend to do things on the spur of the moment without thinking, which can get you into trouble.
- You worry about things going wrong (as they have done before) and therefore do not have much confidence in yourself.

Diagnosis

In the UK, ADHD is most often diagnosed in school-age children. This is partly because it is not usually diagnosed before 6 years of age, and also because teachers tend to pick up on behavioural problems when a child is expected to sit still and concentrate on work in class.

Diagnosis in children is made by a psychiatrist, paediatrician or other healthcare professional who has been trained in diagnosing ADHD. Children are usually referred for assessment by their GP or school.

In an assessment, the clinician will want to talk to the girl and her family about their lives and the things that are difficult. They will usually talk to the girl's teachers and might visit the school to observe her in class. Often families and teachers are asked to fill in questionnaires to help clarify how severe the problems are and in what areas there are particular difficulties.

Sometimes ADHD is not picked up in childhood. Adults can be referred by their GP to a psychiatrist or specialist health professional, who will ask questions about the woman's childhood as well as about current problems. They might find it helpful to talk to family members who can remember how someone behaved as a child. They sometimes use questionnaires to gather information about the problems experienced in childhood and adult life.

What can be done to help?

There is no cure for ADHD, but there are treatments that can reduce the symptoms to a more manageable level. Many people find that symptoms improve with age and as they learn better strategies for dealing with symptoms and certain situations. It is estimated that two-thirds of children with ADHD continue to have some symptoms as an adult. Women with ADHD who receive the right support and treatment are usually able to lead a full life and have the potential to do well at school and work just like anyone else.

Treatment

In children, the initial management is specialised parent training to help parents deal with and minimise further problems. Medication can be used in both children and adults with ADHD.

The most commonly used medications are stimulants such as methylphenidate. Stimulants increase the levels of neurotransmitters (chemicals), such as dopamine, in the brain. Some of these medications work for a few hours and need to be taken several times a day; others last longer and only need to be taken in the morning. Because of the potential for misuse of these drugs, they are legally controlled and how they are prescribed is carefully monitored.

Atomoxetine is a non-stimulant medication used when someone cannot take stimulants because of side-effects or health problems, or when stimulants have not worked well. It works by changing the amount of noradrenaline released in the brain.

Medication for ADHD needs to be started by a specialist to monitor the response and any side-effects but, in the longer term, GPs can often continue the prescription and do the necessary checks. We do not know how long people should continue with medication and there is limited information about long-term effects and effects in pregnancy. There should, therefore, be regular consideration about whether the medication is still having significant benefits or not. Women are generally advised to try and come off the medication before becoming pregnant.

Current guidelines suggest that some talking therapies help to reduce ADHD symptoms, especially when used in combination with medication. Cognitive–behavioural therapy (CBT) is recognised as being effective in improving some symptoms. CBT can help individuals build skills to do important tasks, be more organised and reduce negative thoughts and anxiety. It can be done one-to-one or in groups.

Educational and skills training programmes and support groups can be useful in helping to improve understanding of the condition and for learning positive coping strategies to minimise the impact of symptoms and the effect on families.

Tips for a woman with ADHD

Get help

- Find out more about ADHD. There are many self-help books, apps and support websites.
- If you need more support, join an online support group to find other people in your position who can help you and share their own tips.
- Talk to your friends and family about your diagnosis and difficulties so they understand more about what helps and what you find hard.
- Tell your boss, school or college; they might be able to make positive changes to your environment to help.

Get organised

- Set an alarm 15 min earlier than you need to get up to give yourself extra time.
- Set time aside for planning and organising every day.
- Use a wall calendar and place it somewhere you will look every morning, like the fridge door.
- Use the diary and reminders on your phone to help you remember your appointments and other events within the family.

- Consider setting up bills by direct debit as it saves you having to remember when they are due.
- Use brightly coloured sticky notes in visible places (e.g. the front door or by the kettle) to remind yourself about important things.
- Gather all the things you and everyone else needs for the next day before you go to bed and put them by the front door.

Look after yourself

- Take time out – make sure you get time to relax regularly.
- Find ways to let off steam, like exercising or listening to music.
- Avoid things that make symptoms worse (e.g. using alcohol or drugs).
- Get help from friends or family and other sources to give yourself a break.
- Remember there are probably lots of things you are very good at.

Psychotic illness

Alison R. Yung, Kathryn M. Abel and Sarah Cornick

Holly's story

Holly is an 18-year-old student who lives with her mother in an inner-city area. She had been well until about 5 months previously. In spite of being an above-average student, she started having difficulty with schoolwork. She became easily flustered about homework, frequently missed deadlines and cried about how stressed and tired she felt. She started missing school frequently.

Two months later, Holly started having aches and strange feelings all over and inside her body. She started hearing indistinct whispers, which distressed and further distracted her. The whispering gradually became clearer, until she could make out voices telling her she was ugly and really a man. She started to become unsure of her gender, attributing the strange bodily sensations to her changing sex. She later refused to attend school at all and also refused to see the general practitioner (GP).

Holly became increasingly tearful and stopped washing. She locked herself in her room and her GP advised her mother to take Holly to the local hospital for assessment. Holly was subsequently referred to the local community mental health team, which became concerned about her level of distress and the thoughts she was experiencing that life was not worth living. The mental health team identified her as having a psychotic illness and she was admitted to hospital.

Holly had no past history of psychiatric illness and her childhood was uneventful, except that her mother had experienced postnatal depression after Holly's birth. Holly's parents were divorced, but had shared custody. Although Holly had not visited her father for 3 months before admission, she felt she had a loving relationship with both of them. Her personality had been described as 'bubbly and warm' until 6 months before admission, when she had become less happy and more anxious than usual.

Holly was an in-patient for 3 weeks. She was treated with antipsychotic medication. She also received a sleeping tablet at night for a short period after her admission and underwent tests to make sure there were no underlying physical reasons for her symptoms.

Holly settled quickly on the ward and had a good rapport with her treatment team (psychiatrists, nurses, psychologist and occupational therapist). Her level of distress reduced almost immediately, although the delusions and hallucinations persisted until the antipsychotic medication had been established. Following her return home, Holly attended appointments every 4 weeks with a psychiatrist in her community mental health team. Her symptoms continued to lessen and she regained her usual personality. Holly was also allocated a care coordinator who worked with her on stress management and coping strategies.

Several months after discharge, Holly stopped attending appointments and the community team were unable to make contact with her. Eventually, she attended an appointment, and it emerged she had stopped taking her medication and started smoking cannabis. She was again speaking about being a man and had refused to have sex with her new boyfriend because she was unsure of her own sex. She was readmitted to the in-patient unit and antipsychotic medication was restarted, to which Holly responded quickly.

Holly reported that she had not had periods for several months and she was concerned this was because she was not a real woman. She was reassured to find out this was a side-effect of the medication, which had elevated one of her hormones and caused her periods to stop. She was prescribed a different antipsychotic that doesn't cause this side-effect. She also learned about the risks associated with using substances such as cannabis and the need to identify and manage possible stressors.

Holly is now attending college and making plans to live independently. She has remained symptom-free on the new antipsychotic medication and continues to meet with her community mental health team regularly.

Holly presented with symptoms of a psychotic illness. Women with psychotic illnesses can have 'positive' symptoms (additional symptoms that you would not expect to see in a healthy person, such as unusual thoughts or experiences) and 'negative' symptoms (withdrawal or a lack of a function that you would expect to see in a healthy person). Holly primarily experienced positive symptoms in the form of hallucinations (hearing voices, strange bodily sensations) as well as delusional beliefs about her body changing.

There are different types of psychotic illness and an exact diagnosis can take some time, even years, to be definitively made. This should not stop treatment from starting. Patients are often said to have first-episode psychosis or early signs of psychosis when they first make contact with mental health teams. This allows their treatment to begin and their mental health to be monitored. Eventual diagnoses include schizoaffective disorder, bipolar affective disorder with psychotic features, substance-induced psychosis, delusional disorder and brief psychosis. One of the most commonly known diagnoses is schizophrenia.

Schizophrenia

Schizophrenia is a serious mental illness. You sometimes hear people talking about 'split personality' or referring to something as 'schizophrenic' in nature. Neither of these describes what it is like for someone with the illness. No one is 'split', and suffering with schizophrenia does not mean you change your mind all the time or are particularly mentally confused.

Some women who develop schizophrenia do so in late adolescence or early adulthood. This is a particularly difficult time, as it can disrupt schooling and social lives with peers, and it's a time of life that even healthy teens find hard to negotiate.

Women are less likely than men to develop schizophrenia. For every female with the symptoms, there are two or three males. No one really understands why this is, but it is the same for other problems linked to brain development, such as dyslexia and other learning problems, or attention-deficit hyperactivity disorder (ADHD) and autism.

Girls and women with schizophrenia have a slightly different spread of symptoms compared with men. Women are more likely to have mood symptoms (e.g. low mood, high mood, anxiety symptoms) and paranoid symptoms, but they are less likely to have some of the more debilitating negative symptoms (e.g. poor motivation, difficulty planning tasks, greater sensitivity to the daily demands of life and to life stress, trouble solving problems or thinking abstractly or about many different things at once). Women also tend to be a little older than men when they develop the illness and are more likely than men to have completed some education or training before they become unwell. They might also have more stable lives including children or ongoing relationships, which might mean they can more easily regain independent living skills once they have had treatment for their symptoms.

Causes of psychotic illness

In approximately 3% of women, a physical problem causes the psychotic symptoms (Abel *et al*, 2010). This is called organic psychosis and doctors must rule it out before making a diagnosis of a non-organic psychosis such as schizophrenia. Physical assessment is also important to check there are no other pre-existing illnesses and to help monitor any side-effects of medication. In most cases, the woman will start treatment before a final diagnosis is made, because it is important to manage distressing symptoms as early as possible.

We do not yet know the exact causes of schizophrenia, but research suggests that a combination of genetic, physical, psychological and environmental factors are involved. Schizophrenia tends to run in families. No single gene causing the illness has been found and it is more likely that certain combinations of genes make people more vulnerable to developing schizophrenia. However, having these genes does not necessarily mean that a woman will become unwell.

The illness has been linked to birth complications, bullying in childhood, social deprivation, parental separation, violence and abuse. Recently, there has been a lot of news linking drug use, particularly in teenagers, with schizophrenia. It is certainly the case that people who develop this kind of mental illness are more likely to use alcohol and illicit drugs like cannabis, amphetamines and other street drugs. There is now evidence that drugs, including cannabis, can trigger symptoms of schizophrenia in people who are vulnerable to the illness.

A maternal history of postnatal depression might be linked with difficulties in adequate parenting and neglect, which might influence the child's developing brain. In Holly's case, however, she was bright and performing well at school, and there was evidence of a supportive home environment, despite the parental separation.

Stressful life events such as being made redundant, bereavement or relationship breakdown can be psychological triggers to psychotic illness. In Holly's case, an increase in the volume and complexity of schoolwork might have precipitated the onset of her illness. Alternatively, the illness might have already been developing and simply made it hard for her to cope with the demands of schoolwork. High levels of expressed emotion (hostility, criticism, intolerance) at home can also trigger illness.

Treatment

Early in the illness, women often do well with a combination of education about their illness, family work, and medical and psychological treatments. Many women with this type of illness can be treated in the community, but some might need to have treatment in hospital if they are very unwell.

Holly's treatment involved a 'biopsychosocial' approach. In the initial phase, the focus was on psychosocial intervention, by bringing her into a hospital environment and removing the stressors of home and school. The medical (biological) side of the treatment was sedative drugs for agitation and antipsychotics to treat the hallucinations and delusions. Holly responded quickly and well to these treatments, which is common in a first episode of psychosis and an indicator of a good long-term outcome (Emsley et al, 2007). Holly's symptoms returned when she stopped taking the medication (Robinson et al, 1999) and started to use cannabis. However, she was also experiencing greater stress at the time, as she was back at home and school.

With all medications, including antipsychotics, comes the risk of side-effects. It is important for a woman to have an in-depth discussion with her doctor about possible side-effects, which can include weight gain, hormonal disturbance (as in Holly's case), sedation and abnormal movements. Different medications can be tried if a woman finds that one does not suit her. Women should try to engage fully with their treatment plans, and can ask for an advocate to support them if they have difficulty communicating their point of view to mental health professionals.

A third of women who develop symptoms of schizophrenia will completely recover, a third will improve to a less severe, remitting illness, and a third will experience a severe course of illness, which can be more disabling in the long term. The odds are that they will at least improve, and women should plan for recovery.

Particular concerns for women with psychosis

Physical and sexual health need special attention in women living with psychosis. Most women with psychotic illness are in their reproductive years and some will be mothers. It is important that these aspects of their lives as women are not neglected. This means they need to feel they can continue to care for their reproductive and sexual health. Having a psychotic illness doesn't mean that a woman shouldn't become a mother, but the stress and hormonal changes associated with pregnancy and childbirth can increase the risk of relapse. It is therefore important for a woman to discuss pregnancy with her doctor, so that supportive plans can be put in place. The discussion will prompt a review of her medication to ensure it is safe during pregnancy, and she will need advice about the safety of breastfeeding while taking medication.

Women with severe and enduring mental health problems have often been the victims of violence and abuse and are vulnerable to unwanted pregnancy, unwanted sexual advances, rape and other forms of exploitation. They are less likely to have health screenings, such as cervical screens, and are more likely to develop sexually transmitted illnesses. Women with schizophrenia are also more likely to be offered long-term contraception, have problems with menstruation or become infertile. Mental health services have not prioritised this aspect of women's health, especially in the context of serious mental illness. But a woman who does not have regular periods across her reproductive years is more likely to experience later problems with heart and bone disease because of a lack of normal female hormones. Having frank and open discussions about these aspects of health early on in care planning encourages a more holistic approach to recovery.

Family and carers

Family work is particularly important in psychosis. Family members often experience guilt and trauma at the time of the first episode (Addington *et al*, 2003). Family members need to acknowledge that this reaction is normal and understand that they are not to blame. Doctors should particularly explain about the non-specific nature of the early phase of psychotic disorders (Yung & McGorry, 1996; Hafner *et al*, 2005), as it can be difficult to recognise an emerging disorder in this phase. Symptoms might resemble those of other illnesses, such as depression and anxiety, or even ordinary adolescent angst. Changes in mental state can develop gradually and, therefore, families, teachers and colleagues often don't notice them. They shouldn't feel blame or guilt for this.

References and further reading

Abel KM, Drake R, Goldstein J (2010) Sex differences and schizophrenia. *International Reviews in Psychiatry*, **22**, 417–428.

Addington J, Coldham E, Jones B, *et al* (2003) The first episode of psychosis: the experience of relatives. *Acta Psychiatrica Scandinavica*, **108**, 285–289.

Emsley R, Rabinowitz J, Medori R (2007) Remission in early psychosis: rates, predictors, and clinical and functional outcome correlates. *Schizophrenia Research*, **89**, 129–139.

Hafner H, Maurer K, Trendler G, *et al* (2005) The early course of schizophrenia and depression. *European Archives of Psychiatry and Clinical Neuroscience*, **255**, 167–173.

Robinson D, Woerner MG, Alvir JM, *et al* (1999) Predictors of relapse following response from a first episode of schizophrenia or schizoaffective disorder. *Archives of General Psychiatry*, **56**, 241–247.

Yung A, McGorry PD (1996) The prodromal phase of first-episode psychosis: past and current conceptualizations. *Schizophrenia Bulletin*, **22**, 353–370.

Postnatal depression and postpartum psychosis

Lucinda Green and Liz McDonald

Postnatal depression

Susan's story

Susan, a 27-year-old single mother, had an unplanned pregnancy. She was worried about how she would cope with another baby. She had recently left her partner because of domestic abuse. Six weeks after her baby was born, she started to feel low, was unable to get to sleep and lost her appetite. She had less interest in her children and found everything a struggle. She felt guilty that she did not love her baby. She considered taking an overdose but did not want to harm herself because there was nobody else to look after her children.

Her health visitor asked her how she was feeling, but she was scared to tell her – she thought it would show she was a bad mother and that her children would be taken away. When she took her baby to her general practitioner (GP), she burst into tears and told the GP how she felt. The GP referred her to a psychologist and her health visitor invited her to a support group for mothers with postnatal depression. She found this really helpful and gradually recovered.

Postnatal depression (PND) is an illness that affects 10–15% of women who have a baby. It often starts 1–2 months after birth, but can begin several months later. For a third of women with postnatal depression, their symptoms start in pregnancy.

Some women feel ashamed or guilty about feeling depressed when everyone expects them to be happy about having a baby. PND is nobody's fault. It can happen to anyone. Having a baby is one of the biggest life changes women experience and can be stressful. Women often feel under pressure to live up to their own or others' expectations.

There are many causes of PND; previous mental illness, lack of support, previous abuse, domestic abuse, stressful life events (e.g. relationships ending) and physical illness (e.g. underactive thyroid) can all contribute. Many different mental health problems can affect women in pregnancy and after birth, not just PND. It is important to get the diagnosis right so that the right treatment can be obtained.

Signs that you might have PND

Symptoms of PND usually last for at least 2 weeks and include:

- feeling low and/or irritable most of the time
- difficulty sleeping, even when the baby sleeps
- poor appetite or comfort eating
- loss of interest and enjoyment in things
- lack of interest in the baby (or your other children)
- negative thoughts (e.g. 'I'm not a good mum')
- feeling guilty and blaming yourself
- loss of confidence
- believing you cannot cope
- not wanting to see people
- feeling hopeless or that life is not worth living
- suicidal thoughts or self-harm
- anxiety symptoms (e.g. fear that the baby will be harmed or die)
- psychotic symptoms (e.g. hearing voices; this can happen in the most severe cases and means help should be urgently sought).

Most women with PND can still care for their babies. However, women with severe PND might struggle to look after themselves and their children. PND can also mean a mother will not feel close to her baby. She might feel guilty that she doesn't feel the way she expected to. A depressed mother often worries about harming her baby. In spite of having these feelings at times, most mothers never act on them. If you do feel like this, tell someone so you can get help.

Treatment

Sometimes women worry about seeking help, fearing they will be judged negatively, or that their children will be taken away. However, GPs, health visitors and midwives have seen many women with PND. They want to make sure all women get the right help and support so they can enjoy and care for their babies.

The help needed depends on how severe the illness is. For mild PND, self-help strategies and support from family and friends might be enough. For those who are more unwell, GPs and health visitors can offer treatment and support. For those with severe PND, treatment from a mental health team might be needed. The good news is that women usually recover quickly and fully with treatment.

Psychological (talking) therapies

It can be a relief to talk to someone about how you feel. It can also help you to understand and make sense of your difficulties. Ask your GP about local psychological therapy services and different types of talking therapy. Health visitors can offer counselling at home in some areas.

Medication

For severe depression, or if talking therapy has not helped, women might need to take an antidepressant. Breastfeeding can be continued while taking most antidepressants.

To decide whether to breastfeed when taking medication, think about:

- how severe the illness is (or has been previously)
- treatments that have helped before
- side-effects
- up-to-date information about individual medications in breastfeeding
- the benefits of breastfeeding
- how untreated illness might affect the baby.

If the prescribed antidepressant makes breastfeeding impossible, remember that the most important thing for the baby is that his or her mother gets better.

Hormonal treatments and alternative remedies

There is little evidence that hormonal treatments work. They can increase the risk of thrombosis. Although many people assume that herbal medicines are all harmless, some (e.g. St John's wort) are not necessarily safe in breastfeeding.

Tips for new mothers who feel depressed

- Tell someone how you feel – your partner, a relative, a friend, your health visitor or GP.
- Sleep or rest when you can. Ask for help with night feeds.
- Do something enjoyable or relaxing (e.g. go for a walk, listen to music).
- Go to postnatal support groups or use online support forums; talking to other women who feel the same way can help.
- Let others help with housework, shopping and childcare.
- Exercise regularly.
- Look at self-help books and websites.

Tips for family and friends

- Listen and offer encouragement, reassurance and support.
- If the mother talks about not wanting to live or about harming herself, or if you think she might have postpartum psychosis, seek help urgently.
- Encourage her to get help and treatment.
- Offer practical help – baby care, shopping, cooking or housework.
- If you are the father, make sure you have some support. Fathers can also get depressed after the birth of a baby. This is more likely if the mother has PND.

Postpartum psychosis

Jamila's story

Jamila, a 33-year-old accountant, was diagnosed with bipolar affective disorder when she was 24, after two psychiatric admissions. She had been well since then and was working until she went on maternity leave. She had a supportive partner and family and was happy to be pregnant. Ten days after birth, after two nights of not sleeping, she started pacing up and down and muttering to herself. She became convinced that her family were involved in a plot to take her baby away. She thought this was being talked about on the news. Her husband found her attempting to jump out of a window, and she said she had to escape as her life was in danger. Jamila was taken to the accident and emergency (A&E) department, from where she was admitted to a specialist psychiatric mother and baby unit.

Postpartum psychosis (or puerperal psychosis) is a serious illness that begins suddenly, most often within the first month after childbirth. It affects about 1 in every 1000 women who have a baby. Symptoms vary and can change rapidly. Women can become extremely unwell very quickly. It can be a frightening experience for women, their partners and family.

Signs you might have postpartum psychosis

Many symptoms can occur in postpartum psychosis. They include:

- feeling 'high'
- low mood, anxiety or irritability
- rapid changes in mood
- confusion
- restlessness and agitation
- racing thoughts
- behaviour that is out of character
- talking more, being more active and sociable than usual
- withdrawing and not talking to people
- not sleeping
- losing your inhibitions
- feeling paranoid and suspicious
- strange thoughts that are unlikely to be true (delusions, e.g. that your baby is possessed by the devil or that people are out to get you)
- seeing, hearing, feeling or smelling things that are not really there (hallucinations).

You might not be able to look after yourself or your baby as well as you normally can. You also might not realise you are ill. Your partner, family or friends might recognise that something is wrong. They will need to ask your GP or the mental health team to see you urgently (the same day), or take you to A&E.

Treatment

Women at high risk of postpartum psychosis

Women who have had a diagnosis of bipolar disorder, schizoaffective disorder or previous postpartum psychosis have a 30% risk of developing postpartum psychosis (Jones & Craddock, 2001). Women might also be at higher risk if they have had another psychotic illness or have a history of psychosis in the family. If a woman's mother or sister had postpartum psychosis, but she herself has not had any previous mental illness, her risk is around 3%.

If you are in one of these high-risk groups, talk to your psychiatrist or GP when you are planning to get pregnant. Of course, not all pregnancies are planned – in that case let your doctor know as soon as possible and also tell your midwife and obstetrician about any current or previous mental illness. Also, tell your mental health team you are pregnant. All these professionals should work together with you and your family to help you make a plan for your care. This might include taking medication (e.g. an antipsychotic) to reduce your risk of becoming ill. You might have an assessment with the perinatal mental health team if there is one in your area. This is a specialist team who care for women with mental illness in pregnancy and up to 1 year after childbirth.

Women with symptoms of postpartum psychosis

Women with postpartum psychosis usually need hospital admission. This should be to a mother and baby unit – a specialist psychiatric unit to which mothers can be admitted with their babies. It will provide support for the mother to care for her baby while she gets the care and treatment she needs. After going home, she will have support from a mental health team in the community. This might be a specialist perinatal mental health team, if there is one nearby.

Most women with postpartum psychosis need medication – usually an antipsychotic, a mood stabiliser or both. It is possible to breastfeed while taking some medications, but often women with postpartum psychosis are too unwell to breastfeed. Women usually fully recover.

Support in caring for the baby

A woman with postpartum psychosis will probably need help caring for her baby – both practical support and help with bonding. Mother and baby unit staff are trained to support women with all aspects of caring for a baby. If a woman does not go to a mother and baby unit, she can get help and support once she leaves hospital.

It is normal to lack confidence in mothering ability after postpartum psychosis. Some women have difficulty bonding with their babies. This can be very distressing, but usually these problems do not last long. Health professionals can provide support in learning how to interact with and respond to a baby. Baby massage and other postnatal groups can be helpful. Health visitors can give one-to-one advice if the woman does not feel up to attending groups with other mothers straight away. Children's centres and voluntary organisations can also help. Most women who have had postpartum psychosis go on to have very good relationships with their babies.

Tips for family and friends

It can be very distressing and frightening to see someone you care about develop postpartum psychosis.

- It is essential you ask for help, as the mother might not recognise she is unwell. If your GP or mental health team cannot visit on the day the symptoms start, take the mother to A&E.
- Make sure you get information about the illness. If this is not available from the psychiatric team then try the Action on Postpartum Psychosis Network (details below).
- Make sure you get some support for yourself. The Network also offers support to partners.
- When the mother comes home, help with baby care, shopping, cooking etc.
- Listen and be as supportive as you can.

Useful resources

Action on Postpartum Psychosis Network
www.app-network.org
Support and information for women who have had a postpartum psychosis, and their families. Online support forum and one-to-one email support from volunteers who have had postpartum psychosis themselves.

Association for Postnatal Illness

www.apni.org

Information and support for women with postnatal mental illness by phone or email from volunteers who have experienced PND themselves.

Family Action

www.family-action.org.uk

Support and practical help for families affected by complex challenges (e.g. mental illness, substance misuse and domestic abuse). Provides various support services, including a perinatal support service with volunteer befrienders.

Home Start

www.home-start.org.uk

Support and practical help for families with at least one child under 5, including help for women with PND.

PANDAS (Pre and Post Natal Depression Advice and Support)

www.pandasfoundation.org.uk

Information and support for women with antenatal depression and PND and for their families. Telephone helpline, email support and local support groups.

Royal College of Psychiatrists

- Information on postpartum psychosis
  (www.rcpsych.ac.uk/healthadvice/problemsdisorders/postpartumpsychosis.aspx)
- Information on PND and related conditions
  (www.rcpsych.ac.uk/healthadvice/problemsdisorders/postnataldepression.aspx)

Tommy's

www.tommys.org

Information about a range of pregnancy-related issues; an excellent section on mental health.

References and further reading

Aiken C (2000) *Surviving Post-Natal Depression: At Home, No One Hears You Scream.* Jessica Kingsley Publishers.

Hanzak EA (2005) *Eyes Without Sparkle: A Journey Through Postnatal Illness.* Radcliffe Publishing.

Jones I, Craddock N (2001) Familiarity of the puerperal trigger in bipolar disorder: results of a family study. *American Journal of Psychiatry*, **158**, 913–917.

Twomey T (2009) *Understanding Postpartum Psychosis: A Temporary Madness*. Prager.

Williams C, Cantwell R, Robertson K (2009) *Overcoming Postnatal Depression: A Five Areas Approach*. Hodder Arnold.

Living longer: normal age-related changes, dementia and depression

Nori Graham and Iracema Leroi

As a society, our concerns about ageing and its effect on our brain have never been greater. With the 'greying' of the population, there is a new focus on the need for a better understanding of dementia and its consequences. This has a particular resonance for women.

- Women live on average about 4 years longer than men.
- Women represent a greater proportion of all the people who develop dementia over the age of 75.
- Compared with men, women more often act as caregivers for those who develop dementia.

Not all ageing leads to disease. Some changes in our cognitive abilities and mental health are part of normal, healthy ageing. As we age we expect not to be able to run as fast, and we should also expect to remember things less easily or accurately than we used to. We should learn to adapt to such inevitable changes.

But it's not all bad news! The ageing brain may bring benefits that are often absent in younger women. In this chapter, we will outline the expected changes in how the brain works with ageing, looking at the impact of the menopause and the possible mental impairment that may affect women in their later years. We will end on a positive note about the benefits of the 'ageing brain'.

Normal age-related changes in cognition in women

As the body ages, so does the brain, and its ability to function reduces. For women about to experience or experiencing the menopause (usually in their 40s or 50s), the ability to remember names, recall recent events and think quickly often becomes more difficult. During this period in their lives, women often complain that their brains are 'fuzzy' or that they are 'losing their minds' as they struggle with their memories. Often described as 'brain fog', this phenomenon has some scientific validity. Research has found that perimenopausal women might have impaired verbal memory and speed of thinking. Luckily, such changes can improve and by the time the women are fully postmenopausal, their cognitive profile may be no different from that of men of a similar age.

But the question remains as to whether this effect is due to changes in oestrogen levels associated with the perimenopause and menopause, or other menopause-related symptoms, such as sleep changes, so-called 'vasomotor' changes like hot flushes and changes in mood (depression and anxiety).

A recent study of over a thousand mid-life American women found that, contrary to expectations, perimenopausal symptoms, such as sleep disturbance and other physical symptoms, could not account for the cognitive changes observed with the perimenopause. Instead, the study revealed that changes in speed of thinking were related to depression and that the rate of new learning was negatively affected by anxiety symptoms. Anxiety may affect cognitive performance by using up 'cognitive resources' and impairing attentional processes that are needed to concentrate and take in new information. We already know that depression and anxiety make it harder for the brain to focus on tasks of cognition, such as problem-solving and decision-making, to the extent that, in elderly people, depressive episodes may mimic the full dementia syndrome. Until recently this has been termed 'pseudodementia'.

Can anything be done to prevent these cognitive and emotional changes? Answers are only starting to emerge and it appears that rather than preventing the changes, it is better to try and manage them.

Some studies point to the benefits to the brain of exercise, eating a healthy, low-fat diet with plenty of fruits and vegetables, and controlling vascular risk factors such as smoking, alcohol intake, high blood pressure, obesity and high cholesterol levels. 'Brain training' exercises, so long as they continue to offer a challenge to a person, can also be of benefit, particularly games which challenge the individual to continue 'moving up a level' of difficulty. So, once you've mastered the 'quick' crossword, try out the 'cryptic'!

Arguments over the pros and cons of using hormone replacement therapy (HRT) continue. The precise combination of hormones and the age of the woman when she starts taking them are likely to be important in determining their precise effects. Many women use HRT to control symptoms of the menopause and to prevent osteoporosis and dementia. The beneficial effects of HRT on brain cognition related to the perimenopause are unclear, but current research suggests that when taken for at least a year, HRT may in fact increase the risk of dementia, if women over 65 years start the combined form (oestrogen combined with a progestogen). Starting HRT much earlier may produce different outcomes, but not enough research has been done on safety, or the risks and benefits, to make recommendations about its use then.

May and Felicity's stories

May is 85 years old. She suffers from moderately severe dementia. She lives at home with her widowed daughter, Felicity, now 63 years old. Felicity gave up her job as an NHS manager 2 years ago to look after her mother, when it became clear May would have to go into a home if she had no one living with her.

Felicity has a long and proud record as a carer. Her father left the family when she was 13, and from then on she helped her mother bring up her two younger brothers. She went to work at 16, but continued to help with the boys. When she married at 23, she gave up work, but soon had two children of her own to care for. With little help from her husband, she did not return to work until the youngest started at secondary school. Multi-tasking again, because the housework and shopping still needed to be done, she became a ward clerk, well known for her conscientiousness, but unambitious.

When Felicity was 50, her husband died suddenly of heart disease. Previously, he had paid all the bills and made all the financial decisions. She now had to do all this herself and manage on a much smaller income. Her friends said she had had a change of personality. She began to apply for more senior positions and was promoted into hospital management. She had been rather retiring in her husband's company, but now she became more socially active, developing a circle of friends of her own, many of them women like herself, widowed or divorced. She loved singing and joined the hospital choir, soon taking over its management.

When she was 61, she gave up work to look after May. She now goes out two evenings a week, once to choir and once to visit friends. Her 17-year-old granddaughter, who lives up the road, comes to be with May when Felicity goes out, beginning her career as a carer early in life. Many years ago, May came and looked after her granddaughter when a babysitter was needed. Felicity still manages the hospital choir, which she can easily do from home. With looking after her mother, managing the choir and making ends meet on the small pension she has at her disposal, her multi-tasking abilities are stretched to the full.

Patricia's story

Patricia is a 72-year-old married woman who has lived in the same home since her marriage to Jed at the age of 23. She enjoyed her life as a homemaker and raised three children before taking up a part-time job at a local flower shop at the age of 53. She liked her job and performed well. She spent her leisure time managing her home, shopping and bowling with friends on a Friday night. After 12 years on the job, Patricia started to notice that she had some trouble processing the flower shop orders. She had to write down all the messages she took by phone, and if she didn't keep herself very organised, she would lose track of her orders. Her boss did not notice at first, but after Patricia made a significant error with an order, it became clear that she was no longer coping with the job.

Patricia became increasingly anxious and tearful, and she lost weight. Her sleep was disrupted. The harder she tried, the more errors she would make. One day she lost her way home and a passerby had to phone Jed to pick her up. Her home life started to suffer as well, and her children and grandchildren became concerned. Patricia eventually left her job and agreed to see her GP. Her GP diagnosed her with late-onset depression and prescribed an antidepressant. She initially responded well to this and her mood picked up. However, after 8 months, she started to have trouble managing the household chores and could no longer go shopping alone. She would forget what she needed. Her speech became increasingly repetitive and she relied more and more on Jed to make decisions about their daily life. Her GP referred her to a memory assessment centre. She underwent memory testing, had a physical exam and brain scan. She was diagnosed with probable Alzheimer's disease and treatment was prescribed.

The stories of May, Felicity and Patricia illustrate a number of ways in which mental health can affect women's lives and in which their lives can affect their mental health.

Dementia in older women

Dementia is a disease of the brain. It occurs with increasing frequency with age, so that it affects about 1 in 6 women by 80 years of age. Early symptoms are increasing forgetfulness, loss of a sense of time, loss of interest and concentration, difficulty in making decisions and odd behaviour. As the disease progresses, women with dementia have difficulty understanding what is said to them, do not recognise their nearest and dearest, need help with eating, dressing, washing and going to the toilet, and become totally dependent on others to meet their needs.

If such care is not available at home, women with dementia need residential care in a nursing home. Because women tend to live longer than men, these homes have a much higher percentage of women living in them. Both at home and in residential care, carers are much more likely to be women, too (Graham & Warner, 2011).

There are two main types of dementia: Alzheimer's disease and vascular dementia. The most common dementia is Alzheimer's disease, the cause of almost two-thirds of dementias. Below the age of 90, women and men suffer equally from Alzheimer's disease, while over 90 it affects more women. Women tend to live with dementia for longer than men. Women suffer from vascular dementia less often than men in all age groups (Ruitenberg *et al*, 2001).

Other types of dementia exist, but are less common. There is no known cause of Alzheimer's disease and, at this stage, we cannot prevent it. Vascular dementia is a disease of the blood vessels supplying the brain. Like other forms of blood vessel disease, such as coronary heart disease, healthy eating and exercising regularly make it less likely to happen. There is no cure for either form of dementia, but in some women medication can temporarily slow its progression. For this reason, it is important that women who are concerned about their memory or cognitive function seek medical assessment early. In some cases, problems in thinking may have reversible causes and are not due to dementia.

Depression in older women

The symptoms of depression in older women are similar to those occurring at other ages (see Chapter 18). The special features of depression in older women result from their social situations and the stresses they have to face. Felicity's story illustrates some of these stresses, and also the protective factors that help to explain why many women are resilient and do not become depressed, even though they may have hard lives.

In her childhood, Felicity had been somewhat protected from the depressing effects of separation from loved ones by the way she and her mother had coped together with her father's absence. Then, as a young woman, there was an expectation that she would combine housework with a job, and she did. As for many women of her generation, it was assumed that Felicity would give up work when she had children, so when her husband died she was in a poor financial position. When she retired, her pension was small, as she had only worked for 20 years (Saunders, 2013).

Resilience to depression

Despite her poor financial position, Felicity did not become depressed. Her progression at work, active lifestyle, circle of friends and acknowledged value as a caring daughter, loving grandmother, loyal friend and choir administrator maintained her self-esteem and protected her from developing a depressive disorder. She was certainly not suffering from loneliness, a strong risk factor for depression (Huxhold *et al*, 2010). Older women suffer from higher rates of depression than older men but, in spite of the stresses they face, most do not become depressed (Piccinelli & Wilkinson, 2000).

Young & Schuller (1991) have described how women, when made redundant, are more able to pick up other threads of activity and maintain their self-worth, compared with men. The authors suggest that women have often had to:

> 'knit together different strands, especially their two sorts of work, whose rewards may be monetary or more fundamentally than that, into a more complex whole. This pattern can be likened not so much to a cable as to a swaying cat's cradle of twists and turns and overlaps' (Young & Schuller, 1991: p. 126).

By contrast, for men, work is a single cable that, if cut, sets them adrift in life.

Women generally have better multitasking and social skills than men and these protect most of them from depression, even though they may face financial hardship and other stresses. Felicity's situation was also typical, in that May's two other, male, children were unable to help her when she developed dementia. Her two sons had busy jobs and, rather than give them up to look after her, they encouraged Felicity to sell her home and move in with their mother as her carer.

Felicity's story illustrates the resilience shown by women in adversity. Her strength of personality is characteristic of her gender. Viewing mental health as a positive attribute and understanding how to develop it provides a useful perspective in both prevention and treatment.

Benefits of the ageing brain

While many women complain of losing the cognitive edge as they age, there is increasing evidence that, as we get older, we also become 'wiser' and that this wisdom might compensate, to some extent, for age-related cognitive decline. What does it mean to gain 'wisdom'? There are many definitions of wisdom, but generally wisdom encompasses the ability to see the wider picture, consider situations in shades of grey rather than black or white, make decisions based on experience and careful deliberation, and better consider other points of view. Wisdom allows us to anticipate situations, predict outcomes and perhaps make more efficient decisions (Strauch, 2011). Such cognitive and emotional ability develops with the maturity of age and life experience, and suggests that we should have a more inclusive role for older people in our 'hyper-cognitive' society.

Conclusions

As women age, expected changes, both positive and negative, occur in cognitive and emotional processes. Age is the most important risk factor in the development of dementia, but careful preventive strategies can delay the onset of dementia

Brain health should be as important a focus for women as other aspects of their physical health, particularly as they age.

References and further reading

Graham N, Warner J (2011) *Understanding Alzheimer's Disease and Other Dementia*. British Medical Association.

Huxhold O, Miche M, Schuz B (2010) Benefits of having friends in older ages: differential effects of informal social activities on well-being in middle-aged and older adults. *Gerontologist*, **50**, 471–481.

Piccinelli M, Wilkinson G (2000) Gender differences in depression: critical review. *British Journal of Psychiatry*, **177**, 486–492.

Ruitenberg A, Ott A, van Swieten JC (2001) Incidence of dementia: does gender make a difference? *Neurobiology of Ageing*, **22**, 575–580.

Saunders C (2013) Pot half full? How women lose out when it comes to pensions. *The Guardian* (www.theguardian.com/women-in-leadership/2013/may/01/women-lose-out-on-pensions).

Strauch B (2011) *The Secret Life of the Grown-up Brain: The Surprising Talents of the Middle-Aged Mind*. Penguin.

Young MD, Schuller T (1991) *Life After Work: The Arrival of the Ageless Society*. HarperCollins.

Part V.
Women and treatment

What women want from medication

Ann Mortimer

Emma's story

Emma, a 26-year-old woman, was depressed a year after the death of her newborn son. She had tried the usual forms of counselling and bereavement support, but they had not worked for her, and her general practitioner (GP) had prescribed an antidepressant. Emma remained low in mood, could not enjoy anything or be cheered up, had poor appetite and sleep, difficulty in concentrating and forgetfulness. She did not enjoy her work at a local bank and her partner was becoming frustrated with her ongoing misery. Her GP changed her antidepressant to another drug. A few weeks later, Emma was much improved, and pregnant – something that had not been discussed at the initial appointment, when she still felt guilty and not ready to have another child. After much discussion and consultation, Emma and her GP made the collaborative decision to continue the use of the antidepressant throughout the pregnancy and not to breastfeed. Emma did well and delivered a healthy baby boy.

Over the next few years, Emma had a number of depressive relapses, usually in response to family problems. This included the suicide of a close relative (Emma had an extensive family history of mental illness). Various medications were tried, and eventually a combination of drugs proved helpful. Emma was then able to complete an intensive course of psychodynamic therapy, focusing on her problematic relationship with her mother. Emma was able to change her perspective and as a result became less vulnerable to future episodes of depression. She left the bank and began working as a carer, a new career she loves. She recently weathered a serious cancer scare without any relapse into depression.

Emma's story demonstrates that pharmaceutical treatment can be effective, even in patients with major mental illness, without serious side-effects. Medication and psychotherapy are not mutually exclusive and many women need both, but they will have to be well enough to be able to benefit from psychological treatment approaches. Also required are a flexible approach on the part of the psychiatrist and much persistence on the part of the patient.

On the surface, there would seem to be no reason why women would want anything different from men from the medications they take. Everyone wants treatment to be effective, work quickly and have no side-effects. Treatment convenience is also a concern for most people, with simple once-a-day dosing preferable to taking several medications several times each day. Side-effects and drug interactions are a constant concern for all patients. How a medicine is taken can also be an issue – most prefer oral medicines over injections, unless they are weeks (or preferably months) apart, and topical preparations such as patches or gels might be preferred to swallowing tablets, as (in some cases) they cause fewer side-effects.

However, women can have different preferences to men, regarding medication. Some women are particularly health-conscious and opposed to drug treatment of any kind. In general, women tend to prefer talking therapy or alternative therapies, such as homeopathy. The trouble is that non-drug treatments rarely have the same level of evidence to back up their usefulness as medications, which have all been through extensive clinical trials. Some alternative therapies, such as homeopathy, seem to have no real evidence behind them, apart from the placebo effect (common to all forms of treatment). The placebo effect is a short-lived and partial response that stems from the individual's belief that something is being done. Women who follow vegetarian or vegan diets might object to the beef-derived gelatine present in capsule formulations of their medicine. All these issues can give the psychiatrist and the patient more problems to solve.

Doctors try to discuss possible side-effects with patients, so that the patient can make an informed choice about taking medication (Table 33.1). Unfortunately, this can result in the 'nocebo' effect – when the mere expectation of side-effects causes the woman to experience them. This happens in research experiments, when the patient is told the medication might cause some symptoms, even if an inactive placebo tablet

Table 33.1 Common psychotropic medications and side-effects

Medication class	Common drugs	Common side-effects
Anxiolytics	Buspirone	Dizziness
	Benzodiazepines	Habituation, amnesia, ataxia
	Pregabalin	Drowsiness, gastrointestinal symptoms
Hypnotics	Benzodiazepines	Habituation, amnesia, ataxia
	'Z' drugs	Dizziness, gastrointestinal symptoms
Antidepressants	Selective serotonin reuptake inhibitors	Gastrointestinal symptoms
Mood stabilisers	Lithium	Thyroid dysfunction, thirst, gastrointestinal symptoms
	Sodium valproate	Gastric irritation, weight gain
Antipsychotics	Quetiapine	Sedation
	Aripiprazole	Insomnia (temporary), anxiety
	Atypical antipsychotics	Weight gain, sedation

with no side-effects is given. It is important to remember that side-effects do not occur in every person who takes a medicine, and it is a rare, unfortunate patient who experiences all the possible side-effects of a medication. Most women do not experience most side-effects.

Sedation

A side-effect often disliked more by women than men is sedation. Many women find themselves 'doing it all' rather than 'having it all', and the last thing a busy woman wants is to feel excessively tired and sleepy. Some antipsychotic medications, like olanzapine, are well known for causing both weight gain and sedation. This is unfortunate, because the medication is very effective for symptoms such as hearing voices or paranoia. Night-time dosing, close monitoring of weight, and plenty of education and support about the beneficial effects of diet and exercise can help if no other medication is effective. Alternative medications such as quetiapine or one of the older medications in lower doses might be considered, especially for women of reproductive age who wish to have children.

Weight gain

For most women, weight gain is a particularly unwelcome side-effect. Not only do women tend to be more concerned about body image than men (see Chapter 23), they also generally gain more weight with psychotropic medications than men. Also, they are more likely to develop diabetes as a result of these metabolic side-effects, possibly because women's different body composition and hormones cause them to metabolise medication differently to men. One important example is the medication clozapine, commonly used for treatment-resistant schizophrenia and bipolar disorder. Women taking clozapine have higher blood levels of the drug for the same dose than men. This kind of difference between women and men in the way that their bodies handle medications might partly explain why women have worse side-effects.

Similarly, if women lose or put on a significant amount of weight, or if they take up or stop smoking, the level of a medication in the bloodstream can change. Smoking clears medications more quickly from the body. By contrast, body fat stores medications. This is important when stopping psychotropic medications, because women tend to have more body fat than men. This means that even after a woman stops taking a medication, it will continue to be gradually released into the bloodstream from the fat tissue for a time.

Significant weight gain not only affects a woman's confidence and self-image, but can also interfere with her fertility and health and the baby's health during pregnancy.

Reproduction

Women's reproductive needs affect their requirements for medication. Some medications can affect reproductive function. Conventional antipsychotics can work as very good oral contraceptives or, in the case of long-acting depot formulations, injectable contraceptives. They block the function of a brain chemical called dopamine, and one of the effects of this is to cause the brain to produce more prolactin, the breastfeeding hormone. In this way, the body is fooled into thinking it is nursing an infant and reduces the chances of pregnancy. Periods can stop and some women actually start producing milk. Some of the newer antipsychotics (e.g. quetiapine, olanzapine and aripiprazole) do not raise prolactin levels.

Sodium valproate is a commonly used medication that should be avoided in women of reproductive age, as it can contribute to polycystic ovary syndrome (irregular or no periods, infertility, hairiness and weight gain).

A major worry for female patients and their psychiatrists is pregnancy. Many women stop taking (or decide not to start taking) medication while trying for a baby, to prevent the unborn child being exposed to these medications during early development in the womb. There is little information about this risk, but most research suggests that the risk to the fetus is very small. Abruptly stopping medicines that control symptoms is not a good idea, particularly for illnesses such as bipolar disorder or schizophrenia. Any woman considering this should discuss it with her clinical team first.

Although every woman is different, there is a high risk of relapse if medication is stopped. If this happens, women are likely to need higher doses to regain control over their symptoms, defeating their purpose in stopping. If a woman and her clinical team weigh up the risks and benefits together, an informed choice can be made. Some medications are an absolute no while a woman is trying for a baby, because their use is associated with known risk of malformations, particularly in the first 12 weeks of pregnancy, which is when the baby's organs and body systems are forming. Sodium valproate (mentioned above in connection with polycystic ovary syndrome) can cause spina bifida and other abnormalities, and lithium can cause heart malformations. Although the risks are small, most women and their psychiatrists consider them not worth taking.

New evidence suggests that selective serotonin reuptake inhibitor (SSRI) antidepressants can cause (rare) problems with difficulty breathing, which is likely to be mild and transient. However, pregnant women and their doctors might be more reluctant than before to use these medications for depression when there are so many other options available, including psychological therapies. SSRIs have also recently been implicated in later risk of autism, although more studies are needed to confirm this claim.

Useful resource

UK Teratology Information Service (UKTIS)
www.uktis.org
This national resource is for members of the public as well as healthcare professionals, and provides information about all medication taken before and during pregnancy and breastfeeding, including psychotropic medication.

What women want from services: a patient's perspective

Sally Dean

In many respects, the requirements and needs of women within mental health services are not very different from those of their male counterparts. However, the way in which they are perceived and treated can be quite distinct.

My own introduction to psychiatry in the 1970s, at the age of 18, was particularly bizarre. After I took a massive aspirin overdose, a male psychiatrist interviewed me on a ward in a general hospital. I spoke to him about the way I felt about myself and my life. He later approached my parents and asked if I had been dropped on the head as a baby. It was a singularly ignorant and dismissive response that I have, unfortunately, encountered time and again.

In spite of the increase in the number of female psychiatrists and advances in mental healthcare and treatments, the predominant view with regard to female patients often remains paternalistic and outdated. Women's mental illness still tends to be seen, in Victorian terms, as 'hysterical', and self-harm and suicide attempts are frequently criticised as 'attention-seeking' or 'manipulative'.

The archaic assumption that women are the main caregivers for those in their lives can encourage them to ignore their own complex needs. Moreover, services can blame them for their inability to continue in their roles as partners, daughters and mothers. The results for women can be manifold – the children of single parents can be unilaterally removed and adopted, their sense of themselves as failures can be exacerbated, and the coercion they can feel to return to these roles often overrules the need for time to become well.

The expectations placed on women vary according to socioeconomic factors, faith, sexual orientation, disability and ethnicity. However, I believe that there are commonalities that bind women together.

From the onset of menstruation to the cessation of the menopause, women can be at the mercy of their changing hormones. The effects of these can be physical and psychological: mood swings, stomach cramps, heavy blood loss, headaches and irritability can be debilitating before and during menstruation. In addition, the fear of, or desire for, pregnancy can increase the pressures placed on women. The menopause's night sweats, hot flushes, headaches and sleep disturbances can leave women tired, anxious and possibly mourning an aspect of their lives that defined them as female.

The inability of services to acknowledge these aspects of women's lives can lead to misdiagnosis or a failure to treat them adequately. When I was a patient on a psychiatric ward, another patient told staff she was pregnant. They rejected her claim, believing it to be part of her mental illness. When it became apparent that she was in fact pregnant, she was forced to have an induced, late-term abortion – an extremely distressing procedure that was entirely unnecessary, if only staff had listened to her earlier. Another woman's severe mood swings before her period were misdiagnosed as borderline personality disorder. Treatment proved ineffectual until a doctor noticed the relationship between her menstrual cycle and her behaviour.

The side-effects of the majority of psychiatric drugs can affect how women feel about themselves and their bodies. Some psychotropic drugs interfere with the menstrual cycle and fertility. Some antipsychotics cause breast tissue growth and simulate lactation (milk production) in women who aren't nursing. Many can cause weight gain. The latter is particularly undesirable in a society that expects women to be slim and attractive. Services rarely acknowledge the extent to which weight gain can affect women's self-esteem. Indifferent attitudes, or criticism that they are too 'sedentary', make the struggle with unwanted weight even more difficult.

Depression, for example, can severely affect motivation, reducing the likelihood that the affected woman will exercise. The effects of medication and the symptoms of mental illness have to be fully recognised instead of blaming women for getting fat. When I gained over 4 stone (25 kg) while taking lithium, mental health professionals said that I 'didn't look overweight', even though I had become clinically obese. I could not recognise myself in the mirror and walking made my back ache. The detrimental effects of the medication on my physical health were ignored, as were my lowered self-esteem and my sense that I had lost control over everything – including the way I looked.

Similarly, libido side-effects are frequently underestimated, or totally ignored, when they happen to women. I have often wondered why erectile dysfunction is seen as so much more important than a woman's inability to fully enjoy sexual relations. The expectations of a partner can increase both guilt and dissatisfaction in any woman affected by medication in this manner.

I have observed that mental health professionals find intelligent and eloquent women particularly challenging. The same does not seem to be a problem with male patients. An ability to confront, and articulate, is anathema in services which often expect compliance and unreserved acceptance. It would seem that this runs contrary to what women are 'supposed' to be – passive and tolerating without question. I have, on many occasions, been told that I am too intelligent to have a mental illness. This seems to imply that only stupid people become mentally unwell. In reality, anyone can develop a mental illness.

It is sometimes wrongly assumed that my lack of improvement means that I don't want to get better. Being able to understand her mental illness does not necessarily mean that a woman has control over it. There still exists a culture of blame if someone remains mentally unwell over a long period of time. Instead of attempting to explore alternatives, services leave a patient feeling that she has failed, instead of *vice versa*.

It is crucial that mental health services incorporate everything it means to be female into care planning and treatment. If services neglect to address all these aspects, women will continue to feel marginalised, misunderstood and not fully supported.

What do women want from services?

- We want to be asked how we would like to be addressed.
- We want to be treated as a complete individual – not as the sum of our symptoms.

- We want to be viewed within the context of our whole lives.
- We want our distress to be taken seriously.
- We want to be listened to.
- We want any claims we make about abuse (past or present) to be believed.
- We want our physical health to be given the same attention as our mental health.
- We want to be seen as who we are, not what we're 'supposed' to be.
- We want our complaints about unacceptable medication side-effects to be taken on board.
- We want to be able to make informed decisions about the treatment we receive.

What don't women want from services?

- We don't want our thoughts and feelings to be 'pathologised'.
- We don't want our children to be taken away. With support we can continue to care for them.
- We don't want to be viewed as difficult if we express our needs and preferences.
- We don't want assumptions to be made about us.
- We don't want to be judged.
- We don't want to be viewed as culpable if we are having problems with our relationships.
- We don't want to be blamed for not getting better.

That's not too much to ask, is it?

Complementary and alternative therapies

Ursula Werneke

Complementary and alternative therapies are popular all over the world. Some complementary therapies, such as certain herbal remedies and acupuncture, are thousands of years old. But we still know comparatively little about most of them, because systematic research has only become available in the past few decades.

Effective, safe, both or neither?

Some complementary therapies are more effective than others. It is difficult to lay down hard-and-fast rules of what to use, how and when. For instance, herbal remedies come in many varieties, including alcoholic or watery plant extracts or teas. In contrast to most conventional medications, we often do not know the therapeutically active ingredient in a complementary therapy, or even if there is one. This makes it difficult to work out a dose. In addition, the fact that complementary therapies are natural does not automatically mean they are safe. Opium is natural, and so is deadly nightshade. Complementary therapies can have side-effects and interact with other medicines.

Complementary therapies women might use

The number of complementary therapies is so vast that reviewing or even touching on all is beyond the scope of this chapter. We will focus on herbal remedies and supplements, and look at some examples concerning:

- depression
- anxiety and insomnia
- premenstrual syndrome (PMS) and the menopause.

Complementary therapies for depression

The following therapies all target serotonin, a natural 'feel-good' chemical produced by the brain. Remedies targeting serotonin can trigger manic symptoms in some people, so women with bipolar disorder should avoid them. Also, women should not combine such remedies with other antidepressants, because the combination might produce too much serotonin.

St John's wort (hypericum perforatum)

The main use of St John's wort is as an antidepressant. It is also a sleeping aid and a remedy for anxiety. It is one of the few well-studied complementary therapies and there is evidence of its effectiveness in the treatment of mild and moderate depression (Apaydin et al, 2016). However, if a woman is severely depressed or suicidal, she is likely to need conventional medicines. St John's wort is generally well tolerated, but it can interact with many other medications and make them less effective. For instance, St John's wort decreases the effectiveness of the contraceptive pill, so women taking both should take further precautions against pregnancy.

SAMe (S-adenosylmethionine)

SAMe is a naturally occurring compound that contributes to many chemical reactions in the body and facilitates the manufacture of some important chemicals in the brain, including serotonin. Some small studies suggest that SAMe is an effective treatment for depression (Galizia et al, 2016). SAMe can be taken in the form of tablets or injections. SAMe is not formally approved as a treatment for depression in the UK, but is available over the counter from some UK pharmacies and UK-based internet sites.

l-tryptophan/5-hydroxytryptophan

l-tryptophan and 5-hydroxytryptophan are building blocks for serotonin. The remedies fell into disrepute in the 1990s, when they were linked to a serious flu-like illness called eosinophilia–myalgia syndrome that resulted in several deaths. The illness might have been due to contamination rather than the effects of the active ingredient, but since we still do not know, it is better to err on the side of caution and avoid these substances.

Folate (folic acid)

Folate deficiency has been linked to low mood and mood swings, but taking folate on its own does not necessarily improve symptoms of depression. In pregnant women, folate deficiency can prevent the baby's brain and spinal cord from developing properly. The resulting malformations are called neural tube defects. Women who are pregnant or trying to conceive should take a daily folic acid supplement until the 12th week of pregnancy.

Omega-3 fatty acids

Omega-3 fatty acids, contained in fish oils, are increasingly thought to help general well-being. They may be useful in the treatment of depression and mood swings, but the evidence is mixed (Appleton *et al*, 2015; Sarris *et al*, 2016). Omega-3 fatty acids are probably not a substitute for conventional treatments, particularly when mental health problems are severe, but they might be of some help in combination with conventional medicines.

When combining omega-3 fatty acids with other supplements, it is important not to exceed the recommended daily intake for vitamins A and E. A good way to stock up on omega-3 fatty acids is by eating oily fish, such as salmon, tuna and sardines. Of course, eating too much oily fish can also lead to problems, if the fish is contaminated with heavy metals. Women who are expecting a baby or breastfeeding should eat no more than two portions of oily fish a week (NHS Choices, 2017).

Vitamin D

Depression seems to be linked to low levels of vitamin D, but it has not yet been shown that taking a vitamin D supplement makes a difference to depression. Our bodies manufacture vitamin D when our skin comes into contact with sunlight. Other light sources, such as light bulbs, cannot replace sunlight. Vitamin D deficiency can occur when people live in less sunny regions, cover the body completely when going out or stay mainly indoors. People with darker skin require more exposure to sunlight to manufacture vitamin D. Vitamin D can also be gained through some foods containing oil, such as oily fish, cheese and eggs.

Remedies for anxiety and insomnia

Valerian, passion flower, chamomile, lavender and hops are traditional remedies for poor sleep and anxiety, but little medical research on them is available. This does not mean they do not work, but at the moment we have little evidence that they do. Kava, an anti-anxiety remedy, is effective, but is unfortunately unsafe, as there are concerns about it causing serious liver problems.

Remedies for PMS and menopause

Phytoestrogens

As both PMS and menopause are linked to hormonal changes, some try to balance the hormones by using similar plant-based substances, known as phytoestrogens. Phytoestrogens are found in soy, red clover, flax seed oil, dong quai, chasteberry and black cohosh. However, there is little research on phytoestrogens and we do not know how effective they really are.

Phytoestrogens are not without risks, since they can stimulate cell growth in tissues. Women who have a history of or genetic risk for breast cancer should avoid such remedies. Some phytoestrogens can interfere with blood thinners such as warfarin, increasing the risk of bleeding. There have been cases of severe liver toxicity reported with black cohosh.

Calcium

Women with low calcium intake seem to be at a higher risk of developing PMS. Taking 1200 mg of calcium daily seems to improve symptoms of PMS. Some calcium will already be taken in with food, and supplements can make up the rest. Guidance suggests that taking up to 1500 mg calcium in the form of supplements is unlikely to cause adverse effects (Department of Health, 2012; Mayo Clinic, 2014). Vitamin D is necessary to keep calcium levels stable and so might also help to improve PMS symptoms. However, we know less about its impact on PMS. Calcium and vitamin D might also prevent or treat bone loss (osteoporosis), which is an issue during menopause.

Other remedies commonly used for PMS

Magnesium, vitamin B6, vitamin E, chasteberry and ginkgo are popular remedies for PMS. However, we are less sure about their effectiveness. For all such remedies, it is important to remain within the safe levels of daily intake to avoid adverse effects. For instance, vitamin E supplementation has sparked a safety debate, particularly for women with heart disease. Vitamin B6 can cause nerve damage at even moderate doses. Evening primrose oil is another remedy that many women use, but there is little evidence that it is effective.

Using complementary and alternative therapies safely

Women who wish to try complementary and alternative therapies should always consult a reliable and knowledgeable health professional. This is particularly important for women who are pregnant, trying to conceive, breastfeeding or taking prescription medications.

In general, high-dose supplements and vitamins seem to do more harm than good. They should be avoided, unless a doctor prescribes and supervises their use. For most severe mental health problems, complementary therapies cannot replace conventional medicines. Keeping an open mind about all options will go a long way towards getting the best treatment results.

Useful resources

Mayo Clinic
www.mayoclinic.org
For useful information, search for 'complementary alternative medicine' on the Mayo Clinic's website.

NHS Choices

- Healthy eating
  (www.nhs.uk/LiveWell/Goodfood/Pages/
  goodfoodhome.aspx)
- Women's health for those aged 18–39
  (www.nhs.uk/LiveWell/Women1839)
- Women's health for those aged 40–60
  (www.nhs.uk/LiveWell/Women4060/Pages/
  Women4060home.aspx)
- Complementary and alternative medicine
  (www.nhs.uk/livewell/complementary-alternative-
  medicine/pages/complementary-and-alternative-
  medicine.aspx)

Quackwatch

www.quackwatch.com
A guide to quackery, health fraud and making intelligent decisions, operated by Dr Stephen Barrett.

Royal College of Psychiatrists

- Eating well and mental health
  (www.rcpsych.ac.uk/healthadvice/problemsdisorders/
  eatingwellandmentalhealth.aspx)
- Complementary and alternative medicines
  (www.rcpsych.ac.uk/healthadvice/treatmentswellbeing/
  complementarymedicines2.aspx)

References and further reading

Apaydin EA, Maher AR, Shanman R, *et al* (2016) A systematic review of St John's wort for major depressive disorder. *Systematic Reviews*, **5**, 148.

Appleton KM, Sallis HM, Perry R, *et al* (2015) Omega-3 fatty acids for depression in adults. *Cochrane Database of Systematic Reviews*, **11**, CD004692.

Department of Health (2012) *Manual of Nutrition*. TSO (The Stationery Office).

Galizia I, Oldani L, Macritchie K, *et al* (2016) S-adenosyl methionine (SAMe) for depression in adults. *Cochrane Database of Systematic Reviews*, **10**, CD011286.

Mayo Clinic (2014) *Premenstrual Syndrome (PMS): Alternative Medicine*. Mayo Clinic (www.mayoclinic.org/diseases-conditions/premenstrual-syndrome/basics/alternative-medicine/con-20020003).

NHS Choices (2017) *Vitamins and Minerals*. NHS (www.nhs.uk/Conditions/vitamins-minerals).

Sarris J, Murphy J, Mischoulon D, *et al* (2016) Adjunctive nutraceuticals for depression: a systematic review and meta-analyses. *American Journal of Psychiatry*, **173**, 575–587.

Contributors

Editors

Kathryn M. Abel is a Professor of Psychological Medicine and Director of the Centre for Women's Mental Health (CWMH) at the University of Manchester.

Rosalind Ramsay is a Consultant Psychiatrist working in adult mental health services at the South London and Maudsley NHS Foundation Trust.

Authors

Gwen Adshead is a Consultant Forensic Psychiatrist at Ravenswood House, Southern Health Foundation Trust.

Roxane Agnew-Davies is a Director of Domestic Violence Training Ltd and an Honorary Research Fellow in the School of Social and Community Medicine, University of Bristol.

Annie Bartlett is a Professor of Offender Health Care at St George's, University of London.

Kamaldeep Bhui CBE is a Professor of Cultural Psychiatry and Epidemiology at Queen Mary University of London and the Head of Department at the Centre for Psychiatry. In 2017, he was awarded a CBE for services to mental health research.

Paul Blenkiron was named Psychiatric Communicator of the Year at the Royal College of Psychiatrists Awards in 2016. He is a Consultant Psychiatrist in York and an Honorary Reader at the Hull York Medical School.

Jed Boardman is a Consultant Psychiatrist and Senior Lecturer in Social Psychiatry. He is the Lead for Social Inclusion at the Royal College of Psychiatrists.

David Castle is the Chair of Psychiatry at St Vincent's Health Australia and the University of Melbourne.

Alys Cole-King is a Consultant Liaison Psychiatrist at Betsi Cadwaladr University Health Board and Clinical Director at Connecting with People and Open Minds Health.

Lisa Conlan is a Consultant General Adult Psychiatrist with the South London and Maudsley NHS Foundation Trust.

Irene Cormac is an Honorary Consultant Forensic Psychiatrist at Rampton Hospital in Nottinghamshire and the past-President of the Royal Society of Medicine's Psychiatry Section.

Sarah Cornick works for the South London and Maudsley NHS Foundation Trust as a Consultant Psychiatrist in a community team caring for patients with psychotic illnesses.

Helen Crimlisk is a Community Consultant Adult Psychiatrist and the Deputy Medical Director at Sheffield Health and Social Care NHS Foundation Trust.

Jennifer Davies-Oliveira is a second year Specialty Trainee in Obstetrics and Gynaecology at the University Hospital of Wales, Cardiff, UK.

Sally Dean is a service user who has had mental health problems since childhood. She is passionate about the improvement of secondary mental health services and the elimination of stigma and discrimination.

Lynne M. Drummond has been a Consultant Psychiatrist and Senior Lecturer with South West London and St George's Mental Health NHS Trust since 1985. .

David T. Evans OBE is a National Teaching Fellow of the Higher Education Academy and a Senior Lecturer in sexual health at the University of Greenwich.

Leila Frodsham has dual training in obstetrics and gynaecology, in which she has worked as a consultant for 8 years, and psychosexual medicine, of which she is Lead for the service at Guy's and St Thomas' NHS Foundation Trust (GSTT).

Nuri Gené-Cos is a Consultant Psychiatrist and Lead Clinician at the Trauma and Dissociation Service of the Maudsley Hospital.

Nori Graham worked for many years in the NHS as a psychiatrist for older people. She is now an Emeritus Consultant in Old Age Psychiatry at the Royal Free Hospital, London.

Lucinda Green is a consultant perinatal psychiatrist at St Thomas' Hospital, London. She specialises in the care of pregnant and postnatal women who have a severe mental illness.

Julia Head has been a Specialist Mental Health Chaplain in the NHS for over 20 years. She is also a transpersonal therapist, and has published widely on the spirituality/religion and mental health interface.

Louise M. Howard is a Professor of Women's Mental Health at King's College London and an honorary consultant perinatal psychiatrist at the South London and Maudsley NHS Foundation Trust.

George Ikkos is the Lead Consultation Liaison Psychiatrist at the Royal National Orthopaedic Hospital, and an Honorary Fellow, Honorary Archivist and former Honorary Treasurer and Chair (London Division) of the Royal College of Psychiatrists.

Chetna Kang is a Consultant Psychiatrist, broadcaster and priest in the Hindu tradition of Bhakti Yoga.

Iracema Leroi is a clinical academic in the Department of Neuroscience and Experimental Psychology at the University of Manchester and a practising geriatric psychiatrist in an NHS Memory Assessment Clinic.

Susan Lingwood is a Consultant Liaison Psychiatrist at North Middlesex University Hospital.

Sally Marlow is a Public Engagement Fellow at the Institute of Psychiatry, Psychology and Neuroscience at King's College London.

Liz McDonald is a Consultant in Perinatal Psychiatrist who is past Chair of the Perinatal Faculty at the Royal College of Psychiatrists, Chair of the Pan-London Perinatal Mental Health Clinical Network and Clinical Lead for training perinatal psychiatrists at the Royal College of Psychiatrists.

Helen Minnis is a Professor of Child and Adolescent Psychiatry at the University of Glasgow.

John Morgan is a Consultant Psychiatrist and eating disorder specialist based in Leeds and London.

Ann Mortimer is an Emeritus Professor at the University of Hull and Consultant Psychiatrist at NAViGO.

Zenobia Nadirshaw is a Consultant Clinical Psychologist with over 40 years of clinical and management NHS experience of health and social care services in learning disabilities and mental healthcare, a professor of psychology and an external examiner to three universities.

Trish O'Donnell is a Development Manager for sexual abuse at the National Society for the Prevention of Cruelty to Children (NSPCC).

Helen Pearce is a Consultant Psychiatrist working within Tees Esk and Wear Valleys NHS Foundation Trust (TEWV).

Raj Persaud is a Consultant Psychiatrist who worked at the Bethlem Royal and Maudsley NHS Hospitals in London from 1994 to 2008, and as an Honorary Senior Lecturer at the Institute of Psychiatry, University of London.

Andrea Phillipou is a Postdoctoral Research Fellow at St Vincent's Hospital, Melbourne.

Sandeep Ranote is a Consultant Child and Adolescent Psychiatrist leading young people's eating disorder services and a director of clinical networks.

Susan Rossell is Director of the Centre for Mental Health and a Professor of Cognitive Neuropsychology at Swinburne University, St Vincent's Health Australia and Monash Alfred Psychiatry Research Centre in Melbourne.

Sue Sibbald is a Peer Support Specialist in Personality Disorders at Sheffield Health and Social Care NHS Foundation Trust.

Gaelle Slater is a Consultant Psychiatrist working in community mental health for Sheffield Health and Social Care NHS Foundation Trust.

Neil Stanley is an independent sleep expert who has been involved in the field for more than 35 years. He began his career at the RAF Institute of Aviation Medicine before moving to the University of Surrey.

Margot Waddell is a Fellow of the British Psychoanalytical Society and a Child Analyst.

Gilli Watson is a Consultant Clinical Psychologist. She works in adult mental health services providing individual and group trauma recovery therapies for women with complex mental health difficulties resulting from childhood sexual abuse.

Ursula Werneke is a Consultant Psychiatrist and Associate Professor in Psychiatry at Sunderby Hospital Luleå and Umeå University in Northern Sweden.

Jennie Williams is a Clinical Psychologist. She is committed to promoting gender-informed thinking, policy and practice in mental health and this has shaped her working life as a practitioner, academic and independent trainer and consultant.

Philip Wilson has worked as a general practitioner in Glasgow for 23 years, as well as working as a part-time researcher at the University of Glasgow.

Alison R. Yung is a Professor of Psychiatry and Director of Research for the Division of Psychology and Mental Health at the University of Manchester and an Honorary Consultant Psychiatrist at the Greater Manchester Mental Health NHS Foundation Trust.

Index

Compiled by Linda English